HEALTHY
HEALING

D0950239

CALGARY PUBLIC LIBRARY

OCT   2017

HEALTHY HEALING

A Guide to Working Out Grief
Using the Power of
Exercise and Endorphins

Michelle Steinke-Baumgard

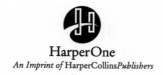

HarperOne
An Imprint of HarperCollins*Publishers*

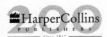

This book contains advice and information relating to health care. It should be used to supplement rather than replace the advice of your doctor or another trained health professional. If you know or suspect you have a health problem, it is recommended that you seek your physician's advice before embarking on any medical program or treatment. All efforts have been made to assure the accuracy of the information contained in this book as of the date of publication. This publisher and the author disclaim liability for any medical outcomes that may occur as a result of applying the methods suggested in this book.

HEALTHY HEALING. Copyright © 2017 by Michelle Steinke-Baumgard. All rights reserved. Printed in the United States of America. No part of this book may be used or reproduced in any manner whatsoever without written permission except in the case of brief quotations embodied in critical articles and reviews. For information, address HarperCollins Publishers, 195 Broadway, New York, NY 10007.

HarperCollins books may be purchased for educational, business, or sales promotional use. For information, please email the Special Markets Department at SPsales@harpercollins.com.

FIRST EDITION

Designed by SBI Book Arts, LLC

Library of Congress Cataloging-in-Publication Data has been applied for.

ISBN 978–0–06–265603–2

17 18 19 20 21 LSC 10 9 8 7 6 5 4 3 2 1

Dedicated to my Addy and Chew, who lit my inner fire when life threatened to extinguish the flame. To my Mitch, who taught me to live in and cherish the moment—your lessons live on. To my father, Quentin, who gave me grit and passion. And to Keith, my man who came after, who showed me my heart was big and wide enough to love again.

Finally, to you, my reader, who have decided it is time to live again. My wish is that this book sets your soul on fire and you do big things with all the days you have left.

You are still here for a reason.

Contents

Message to the Reader

You are not alone. I understand that in many ways you probably feel completely on your own because grief is isolating and the path forward is daunting. Validating those feelings will be part of your healing journey, which starts right now. You've picked up this book, and with that single action you've joined a community of people seeking a positive path forward and a chance to live their best life after loss. While no two grief journeys are ever the same, just knowing you are part of a community will help you survive this time in your life and take active, positive steps forward.

I too have lived in the shadow of loss, and I know the pain, the exhaustion, and the loneliness that accompanies life beyond the death of someone you imagined you couldn't live without. I also know that grief is a very personal experience, one that is as unique to each griever as their fingerprint. *There is no rule book, no set of guidelines, and no time frame to the grief journey.* Loss does not discriminate based on any outside factors—not age, happiness, or health. Loss is universal—the great common denominator. It can certainly come from death (which, as you'll soon discover, was the root of my personal grief story), but through my years working with clients and founding the One Fit Widow community, I've learned that loss comes in many other forms as well and while this book is primarily about loss from death, I'd be remiss if I didn't acknowledge other forms of loss. There is the personal loss of being consumed by a busy life, wondering if you still matter and struggling to find yourself amid your day-to-day tasks. There is also the loss of identity, which can occur in the aftermath of a major life event, such as a divorce or a job loss.

As a child, my father often reminded me that nothing is easy, not for me or any other person who walks this earth. Every time I struggled or failed, my father told me, "Michelle, life is difficult." That phrase came from M. Scott Peck's *The Road Less Traveled*. Mr. Peck brilliantly tells us, "This is a great truth, one of the greatest truths. It is a great truth because once we truly see this truth, we transcend it. Once we truly know that life is difficult—once we truly know and accept it—then life is no longer difficult. Because once it is accepted, the fact that life is difficult no longer matters."[1]

I'd like you to remember the universality of difficult times while you read this book. I want you to remember that challenges are not unique to you and suffering is part of the human condition. *You are not alone.*

There is no question that grief is the most powerful of all emotions—with the exception of love—and if you love in this life, then you will eventually grieve. None of us escapes without shards of glass in our hearts—the darkness, the loneliness that no words can accurately describe. We all experience this pain. However, despite the universality of grief, we've let each other down. We haven't created a healthy plan for healing. In fact, as I argue later in this book, we've done a major disservice to grievers. We tell them to "move on." We try to fit their grief journey into a linear path with arbitrary stages. We force them into unrealistic timelines. We don't give them the tools to start to *feel better.* I hope this book will change that.

While other books and experts are going to tell you the path you must take is to "move on," I'm here to tell you to instead *move forward.* And the best way to move forward is by literally moving forward. Physical fitness is a perfect metaphor for grief—the act of taking steps even when you're tired and feel broken; these are emotional steps you will need to take in your grief journey as well. And as these daily steps forward, even small ones, you will find yourself empowered, strengthened, and walking toward hope.

Shortly after my husband passed, I was on a long run, training for a marathon I would complete in his honor. I remember coming home and feeling solace in the middle of my life's biggest storm. While the hard sweat of my run didn't *fix* my grief, it did allow me to think, breathe, fight, and ultimately process a loss no thirty-six-year-old woman should be forced to handle. That's when I realized fitness is the lifeline so many people are searching for. I realized that fitness is the catalyst that empowers another day; it is a place to just be and offers an opportunity to leave expectations, demands, and stress behind. When you use fitness as an active grief tool and as part of a grief treatment program, like the one you'll find in part two of this book, you will begin to find strength you never knew you had and a new appreciation for life beyond loss. Fitness can and will set your soul on fire—it is that powerful.

At first it may seem hard, but each new step will help drive you forward. I'm not going to promise you that this book or fitness in general will be the answer to your struggles, but I will promise you that if you give it a try, you might just find yourself changed from the inside out. It is my hope that through this book you will lean toward physical exercise and fitness as a powerful coping mechanism for your grief.

Despite the guaranteed pain that comes with life, we would never give up love to save our hearts from grief. We would never walk away from the memories, the joys, and the laughter to not feel the pain on some unforeseen day.

Instead, we all love. We all grieve. We all grow beyond the immediate pain, and we carry the scars in our hearts forever. I'm not without scars and neither are you. That's okay. Scars don't make us broken; they make us beautiful.

Our past has shaped us.

Our past has given us struggle.

Our past has helped us grow into better people.

Our past has shown us the worst moments a life can endure.

But *never* has our past defined our future.

You have free will over all your todays and tomorrows, and while your past may have been full of painful life lessons, your future is full of whatever you want it to be. You have the choice to rise from your ashes and live more boldly, bravely, and beautifully than ever before.

I'm ready to take you on a new journey of healing. Not the kind of healing that pretends to erase the pain, but healing that lets you process the pain, move within the pain, and use the pain to propel your life forward. I'm going to ask you to do your part in creating a new life after loss. I'm going to ask you to move forward physically while moving forward emotionally, all while honoring the life that has taken you this far. It won't be easy, and you will have days when life feels next to impossible, but this is not the end of your journey. This is just the beginning.

Are you ready to come with me? Are you ready to live again? Are you ready to connect to your inner fire?

It's time to start *healthy healing*.

XO,

Michelle

How to Use This Book

This book is not designed to be a typical "grief" book. I've created this book to help you move *beyond* the grief box. While society may tell you that your journey should be neat and organized, I understand that grief is chaotic, and I will empower you instead to take personal responsibility for your path forward.

What I've written is intended to make you think, reflect, question, and grow. Grief will happen, and there is nothing you can do to stop the pain and evolution of your being through this tragic time in your life. Still, you have a daily choice to make, and this book will help you make the choice toward hope and healing.

Please don't mistake the word "healing" in the book's title to mean that I expect you to *heal*. Being completely "healed" is one of the many outdated myths surrounding grief (we will discuss more myths later), but I do believe you can take daily steps in each moment that will help you in your process toward healing. What you've experienced will stay with you and become part of the fabric of your life. Don't deny the colorful tapestry of your new, complex existence. The colors will be bold, rich, and vibrant if you allow them to be.

I've written this book at a time when our society is moving at the speed of light, yet our grief path is stuck in a mold that should have been shattered long ago. Healthy healing entails breaking away from the rules placed on our intricate emotions and from stunted views of mortality. We all live, and we all die. The awakening of our spirit needs to happen in order for us to face the hard truth of death for ourselves or for the people we love.

Because I'm writing this book for this new age, I've designed the Healthy Healing program as an interactive experience. You have the option to become part of a unique online portal designed to help you make the changes and implement the work laid out in the pages you have before you. There, you can view workouts and recipes, interact with other readers, and share your success stories, your struggles, and your personal evolution. You also will be able to hear podcast interviews on all forms of healing, from fitness to nutrition, living beyond loss and learning to embrace less so you can live more. The portal will continue to grow and evolve, just like I've asked you to do in the chapters ahead.

I encourage you to hashtag #healthyhealing via social media whenever you complete a part of the program so other people can find and be inspired by your stories and you can hold yourself accountable for progress.

Connect with me too. I love to interact with my readers, and I want to hear how you have chosen to live a bold new life after whatever loss you have endured.

Interactive portal: www.healthyhealingbook.com/healing

Facebook: www.facebook.com/OneFitWidow

Twitter: www.twitter.com/onefitwidow

Instagram: www.instagram.com/onefitwidow

If you'd like to learn more about me and the exciting work my team is doing to help people live their best lives after loss, you can find more information at

Personal blog: www.onefitwidow.com

Virtual training company: www.my1fitlife.com

Nonprofit organization: www.livethelistnonprofit.org

HEALTHY HEALING

My Story, Your Story

My Story

Sitting on a beautiful beach in Los Cabos, Mexico, I hit my personal rock bottom. I remember sitting there, looking out at the beautiful turquoise sea, and thinking that all I wanted to do was curl up and cry. For the first time in my entire life, I hated myself, and the only one stopping me from changing was me. Like so many mothers, I'd thrown myself into parenting, being a good wife, and of course my corporate job. From the outside looking in, my life was beautiful— society's view of perfection. I had two healthy and amazing children, I was married to my best friend of fifteen years, and I had a dream job that allowed me to travel around the world and see amazing resort destinations. I'd created my own version of the white picket fence, but for some reason it sometimes felt like my personal hell.

For most of my life I'd been thin. Not necessarily healthy, but always thin. (We often equate the two—health and thinness—but nothing could be further from the truth.) After I married Mitch, my lifestyle started to catch up with me. Eventually, with the addition of two babies and a busy corporate job, the pounds started packing on. I put everyone else's needs above my own. I forgot that I mattered, that my life mattered. It's ironic to me now, as I look back with a clear vision and the perspective of loss, just how silly it was to ignore my needs.

My job was paramount in those days. I'd wake up to a mountain of emails, and before my feet hit the floor I'd feel in the weeds and under tremendous stress. My babies were both under three, and my husband had recently gone through a rigorous year of training to live his dream of becoming a professional pilot. The result of my busy lifestyle was a body that was tired, slow, and weak and a soul that was sad, lost, and desperately in need of rest. My lifestyle and habits were making me less productive at work, less satisfied as a wife, and less happy as a mother. During that quiet moment in Mexico I looked at my husband and said, "I can't live like this any longer; I'm miserable in my own body."

He took my hand, looked me in the eyes, and said, "Then fix it. Only you can."

Those words stuck, and while they seemed like common sense, for the first time in my life I realized I had to take personal responsibility for my unhappiness. I was not a victim of my body and the life I had created; rather, I was going to become a victor in the life that lay before me. From that beach resort, I picked up the phone, called a local trainer, and decided it was time to own this life and take charge of my future. From the rock bottom, there is only one way to go, and I was ready and willing to head *up*.

We flew home, and in late August of 2009 I took back the power in my life. I remember walking into the gym for the first time. As they weighed me, took my measurements, and even took my picture, I was mortified. I remember trying to pick out a cute outfit to wear to help hide the fact that I'd let my body get so bad. There was no hiding now; my secret was out, there was work to do, and only I could do it.

At 206 pounds and nearly 40 percent body fat, I had to take charge of my story. I had to write an alternate ending.

Throughout the next month I exercised hard, and within a few weeks I felt like a new person. I quickly lost about fifteen pounds, but more importantly, I gained confidence and strength, and even found more time in each day. My new habits were paying dividends, and I was euphoric with my progress. In early October I flew to Florida for business, and I managed to stay on track despite early-morning meetings and poor food options. I had finally found a place within myself where I was determined not to let any life circumstances derail me from my goals. I'd been faced with challenges in the past, and I'd often joked that if I stubbed my toe wrong, I would quit a fitness program. It had always seemed like the first thing to go when life got tough, but something was different this time. I knew I wasn't going to stop. I was on fire, and there was no quitting now.

I flew home from Florida on October 8, 2009, and my husband met me at the airport with our two-year-old daughter, Addison. If I close my eyes, I can still see them standing there. He was holding Addy in one hand and roses in the other. She ran to me and clung to my leg as he walked over and embraced me with a warm, welcoming kiss. He whispered in my ear, "I'm so proud of you, baby. Way to take control of your life," and I shed a tear. For the first time in a very long time, I was proud of me too. We drove home, where my mother-in-law was staying with our one-year-old son, Matthew, and I quickly went to bed. Tomorrow was a big day with an early workout. I was inspired; life was starting to become everything I had dreamed it could be.

The next morning began like any other typical morning in our lives. I trained at my gym at five A.M., came home, got my daughter ready for preschool, and started my crazy day at work. Mitch was getting ready to leave for a flight interview, and for whatever reason,

I remember taking a mental note of how he looked as he stood at the dining room table and went over his flight log for the morning. He was wearing khaki pants and a white shirt, and even after fifteen years, I still thought, *Man, does he look cute.* My newfound love of fitness had awakened me to so many things that had been missing in my life, even the simple joy of appreciating my husband. As he drove off to take our daughter to preschool, I watched them back out of our driveway, and I waved good-bye. Little did I know that just a few hours later my world would fall apart.

In the early afternoon of October 9, 2009, Mitch took flight in a 1918 S.E.5a replica and crashed shortly after takeoff. At the time, I was working away at my desk, completely unaware of the tragedy unfolding in my blissful life. Soon after two P.M. I drove my daughter to her dance class and began to text her father, who had been planning to meet us. The texts to him went unanswered, so I called his cell phone. The rings went straight to voicemail, and I started to have an uneasy feeling in my gut. He always called or texted me just after landing to assure me all was well. I pushed my fears aside, told myself I was being silly, and went about my day. As I watched our daughter dance, my phone rang, and it was my mother-in-law, who was audibly shaken. All she said was "You need to come home. There has been a plane crash at the Deer Valley Airport, and they fear it might be Mitch." I grabbed my little girl, and we got in the car and started the twenty-minute drive home.

As I drove, I felt as if I were having an out-of-body experience as I detached from the life I was living. I was thrust into the shock in a profound way. The traffic on the freeway was stopped, and my phone rang again, jolting me back to reality. My mother-in-law was on the line, and she told me to hurry up and come home because they were sending someone out from the airport to talk to me. That's when I knew he was gone. If he were alive, they would have sent me to a hospital or the airport, but by their sending me home, my worst fears had been validated. He was dead, and that was all the confirmation I needed.

The exit for the airport was just ahead, and for a brief moment I felt as if I should go to the crash site; I needed to go. Then I looked back at my baby girl in the backseat of my car, playing with her blond curls, smiling in her car seat, and I knew I couldn't take here there. As parents, we have to make hard choices, and at that moment her safety and naïveté were the most important things in my life. She was blissfully unaware that her father may be gone, and I knew I had to go home for her sake and mine. I walked into our home and found my mother-in-law on the floor, completely shattered. I helped her up and calmly said, "Not in front of the kids." There is no adequate way to put into words the power of a mother and wife in the throes of tragedy. We all grieve differently, and my natural instinct was to be strong, powerful, and, yes, distant. I love my mother-in-law deeply. I love my children deeply. I love Mitch deeply. Love was never the question. But our bodies can absorb only so much pain in one heart-breaking moment. My body was overloaded from the top of my head to the tips of my toes.

As we sat in relative silence, waiting for the person to come out from the airport, we watched the clock circle past the hours. The day turned into night, and I felt a disconnect between my body and my spirit. I witnessed the nightmare that my life had turned into, and I questioned everything I'd ever known. I'm a good person. I have a good heart. Bad things don't happen to good people . . . or do they?

A knock at the door stopped my racing heart. I didn't want to answer it because the other side of the door held nothing for me. On the other side of the door was agony, regret, and a lifetime of grief. On the other side of the door was misery, and I was not ready to face the certainty. I took a deep breath and opened the door to my reality. A wave of emotion blew in with the cool October air and with it the energy surrounding death: harshness, loneliness, and horrifying sadness.

An army of people stood beyond the door. There were fire trucks, police cars, men and women in uniform who took their first glimpse of the ladies whose lives they were about to destroy. They looked as stunned as I'm sure I did. A man asked if I was Mrs. Steinke, and I confirmed that I was. He asked if they could come in, and I moved to the side as they all walked past. We settled in the living room . . . all twenty of us. I looked around the room. *Why so many people? What is going on? Is this normal?* The lead investigator introduced himself as well as the local firefighters and two grief counselors. *What the hell? There is no way this is happening. This crazy dream I'm having needs to stop, and it needs to stop right now!* That's when I was given the worst news a wife and mother could ever possibly hear. "Mrs. Steinke, I regret to inform you that the 1918 S.E.5a replica he was flying indeed crashed at Deer Valley a little before two P.M. this afternoon. Was Mitchel planning on taking the plane up?" I replied, "Yes." The investigator said, "I further regret to inform you that we cannot identify the pilot. The damage is too severe." No one is ever prepared to hear words such as those. I just kept hearing the phrase "the damage is too severe."

We sat there in complete silence for what felt like an eternity. The officer pulled a chair up in front of me and got uncomfortably close. He was in my personal space as he held my stare. "Mrs. Steinke, I've been an investigator for twenty plus years. I've made countless calls like this. I've seen families destroyed in the blink of an eye. I need to tell you one critical thing." I could feel his intent, and I could sense his sincerity. I locked eyes with him and returned to my place in the moment. I knew whatever he was about to say I needed to hear. "Michelle, whatever you do, don't drink. Don't numb your pain in *any* way. Live it, experience it, survive it, and you will be okay."

The words "you will be okay" seemed so inaccurate in that moment. I remember thinking *I will never recover from this* and *I will never be okay again*. In that time of anguish, intense sadness, and harsh reality, you don't know what to cling to, what to reach for, or even what your name is. It's like you've been dropped into the deepest and darkest hole, and there's no hint of light in any direction. There are no words in any human language that can accurately depict the pain of grief.

As I lay in my bed that night after being told the father of my children and the love of my life was dead, I could hear the officer's words play in my head again and again: "Michelle, whatever you do, don't drink. Don't numb your pain in *any* way. Live it, experience it, survive it, and you will be okay." His words resonated, and they mattered. He was sent to tell me those words and to have an impact on the path of my grief. In fact, I believe he was sent to change the trajectory of my life forever.

The next morning I walked downstairs and looked at my best friend, Christine, who had come to our house to make calls to family and friends, and I asked her to call the gym. I was participating in a weight-loss challenge, and I felt compelled to finish what I had started. I wanted the gym to know that despite the tragedy unfolding in my life, I would continue my journey to get fit. I didn't know much about my future at that moment in time, but I knew the move I would make next would profoundly shape the remainder of my life. I would not quit on my fitness. Everything inside my being was telling me not to quit. Everything was telling me that *this* was *really important*.

At a time when our lives have been shattered, we all need something that will pull us through. We all need a lifeline that will help us see the light again and help us find the strength to carry on. What I didn't realize at the time was that fitness would be my thing.

Within a week I found myself back in the gym and working out. My workouts quickly became my saving grace—the only thing that helped me feel sane, my outlet for unimaginable grief. In the gym, I felt somewhat normal, and that is a gift to any grieving person. I craved normality, but normality is often fleeting after loss. Fitness gave me a chance to escape the pain for a short time and find a release for all the anger, sadness, and frustration. When I was at the end of my rope as a now solo mother of two tiny babies and as an unexpected widow, I could direct my feelings toward a healthy outlet for my grief and pain. I could fuel my fire to continue living, empower my being, and generate energy at a time when it might have seemed much easier to curl up in bed and drink myself into oblivion. Life had handed me options, and the officer's words just kept playing in my mind over and over again.

In my years since that loss I've never once regretted my choice to use fitness as my strongest grief-coping mechanism. I've never once regretted picking myself up and going to the gym just a few days after Mitch passed and using that time to find my strength in a solid sweat. I've never once regretted showing my children strength when I could have shown them weakness. It was not always easy to make the choices I made, and for many oblivious onlookers, it may have appeared selfish or self-absorbed. Those who have never grieved often feel the need to tell you that you are doing it all wrong, but what I've learned is that there is no shame in a good sweat, just a soul-cleaning power and a release of the pain. No other person will face this journey the same as you do, and therefore they have no right to tell you that you are doing it wrong. This is your life, and you must not numb yourself to the struggles. Live it, experience it, survive it, and you will be okay.

Eventually I found my fitness experience to be so powerful I just knew it had to be shared with the world. Within a year, I left my corporate job to become a fitness coach and went on to launch the blog One Fit Widow. The name was never about me but rather about

redefining a word, "widow," that has had deeply negative conno-
tations in our society. When we hear the word "widow" we think
sad, lonely, dark, and even old. I wanted to breathe power, strength,
and energy into a conversation that screams dark, lonely, and sad.
Grievers come in all ages and from all backgrounds; we can no longer
ignore the vibrancy and brilliance they can bring to the world. The
response was overwhelming. I received countless thank-you emails
and notes telling me it was about time the people who were grieving
felt empowered enough to come out of the shadows and claim their
paths forward, positive and negative, and to do so with strength and a
healthy view on their difficult choices. There are still those who don't
agree with my viewpoint on loss, and that's okay. While I believe we
can all learn from one another, my view is a simple one: just take what
you need and leave the rest.

What has defined my story has been a combination of both my
many failures and my moments of success. I want you to understand
that you define this life, and you are still here for a reason, regardless
of your failures, losses, or triumphs. No matter what happens next,
you have the ability to pick up a pen and write an alternate ending to
your story. You have the ability not just to survive but to thrive.

Your Story

So here you are, faced with options and a story that matters and is
worth sharing. What defines your story is up to you and you alone.
I need you to accept this fact because it is paramount to your success
with the Healthy Healing program. I know that what you are facing
is hard, that the mountain ahead seems too high to climb and you may
be feeling too tired to climb it, but you are here just the same. You
picked this book because you are looking for strength and hope. Both
of these things are already inside you. I want to help you face your

challenges head-on and become stronger, healthier, and more alive than ever before.

What choice will you make with your life after loss?

What Mitch once told me I am now telling you: *Only you can change your life.*

You can't control what has happened in your past, but you can define how you will spend your future. Your grief is now a part of who you are. You are a beautiful and complicated tapestry of life lessons, emotions, and growth. You are changed forever, and you can choose to cope in a healthy and ultimately empowering way or you can choose to numb the pain. I'd like to help you choose healthy healing. I'd like to help you find strength and power through all that you already possess inside you.

Step forward into your future while honoring your past.

Take your grief and allow it to remind you to live.

Never move on but always move forward.

PART ONE

Moving Forward

CHAPTER 1

Myths About Grief

This book is going to offer you a healthy new way to go about your grief journey. But before we get there, it's worthwhile to debunk some of the myths about grief. Recently I wrote an article for the *Huffington Post* called "Stifled Grief: How the West Has It Wrong."[1] It's been one of my more popular articles, I believe, because it provides an accurate view of how grief works and how we try to stifle it culturally. The article resonates with people because it's honest, raw, and vulnerable. It's time for us to stop pretending that grief looks like a neat, organized package and to instead paint it in the colorful light and as the abstract art it truly is. The following are ten of the biggest grief myths I've come to recognize, which we need to dispel before we move into the program.

MYTH 1
Grief Is One Size Fits All

I'm going to let you in on a little secret, something that is not widely accepted in our grief-stunted society: There is no "right" way to grieve. There is no timeline, no five-step program, and no textbook to help you navigate the road ahead. I'd love to tell you differently. I wish I could share a step-by-step guide complete with timelines and flowcharts, but that would be less than honest about the reality of life after loss.

Now I'm going to tell you another secret: There are going to be people in your life who will give you endless advice about taking a year (give or take) to grieve, but after that arbitrary time frame, they will grow tired of your pain, anxiety, and sorrow. You may start hearing rumbles of discontent and hurtful words like "It's time for you to start moving on" or "Shouldn't you be over that by now?" It pains me to tell you this because I know it is the last thing you want to hear. But it is the truth.

What is important is to understand that you need to grieve the best way for *you*. The method for you may be entirely different from what worked for someone else.

Yes, you can be angry. Yes, you can be sad for as long as you need to be. Yes, you can and will be emotionally drained. Yes, you can laugh. Yes, you can even be happy again.

Take each emotion in stride and try not to label yourself, compare yourself, or tell yourself that you're not doing it right. Don't allow others to tell you that either, because grief is an entirely individual experience. Above all else, do what is right for your soul.

MYTH 2

Grief Happens in Stages

Our culture likes to impose ridiculous timelines and expectations on the experience of death, divorce, and other traumatic events. Grief does not look or feel like our expectations; neither does healing. No set of false expectations does grievers more of a disservice than the "five stages." Originally written for those who are facing their own

Healing Is a Journey, Not a Destination

The use of the word "healing" in this book is intentional, though I don't expect you to ever fully *heal* from what you've experienced. I expect that you will absorb your loss and in some way carry it with you forever. The word "heal" sets up a false expectation that there is some magical destination you will someday arrive at where you will feel all better and your loss will no longer affect you. That misconception is outdated and in many ways detrimental to your true healing. Allow yourself a healing process, but don't expect to heal. Expect to change, grow, and evolve instead.

mortality, the five stages theory has mistakenly found its way into the expectations of those who are grieving as well. This model makes grief look like a linear path, one that leads to complete healing as the griever travels somewhat effortlessly from denial to acceptance.

What grief *actually* looks like is less like a straight line—in which you move from stage to stage with ease—and more like the flight plan of a neurotic bee. One moment you are sad, the next you are angry, and still the next you are accepting and peaceful. Grief will take you all over the emotional spectrum and leave you feeling tired, both physically and emotionally. My best analogy for grief is a tsunami wave that sweeps you off your feet with no warning and with tremendous power. The wave is intense and leaves you with no view of the shore and gasping for air. No matter how hard you fight the tide, you are powerless to stop it, so you have no choice but to surrender and ride the wave. Moments of grief will come and go in no particular order and without your consent.

Knowing that your grief journey may feel haphazard and unconventional frees you of the expectation that grief should be a simple transition over time.

MYTH 3

You "Move On" from Grief

A griever hears every platitude in the book: "They are in a better place." "At least they aren't in pain." "God needed them more." People mean well, but most have no idea how little these generic blanket statements help and, in many cases, how badly they hurt.

When I became a widow, no two words cut more than "move on." Those two innocent little words carry a negative connotation for anyone who grieves. They insinuate that there is a "right" way to grieve, placing unfair expectations on someone experiencing loss and causing feelings of inadequacy and panic. The griever is left questioning their methods and their emotions.

When you experience significant loss through death or other traumatic experiences, you absorb the pain, and it becomes part of who you are. It profoundly shapes who you become. There is no moving on from such experiences; there is only moving forward. I know I'm repeating myself here, but this is one of the most crucial elements to my grief program. Moving forward means you haven't forgotten your loss or the future you'd planned before death stole it from you. Moving forward means you have chosen to continue living while remembering what came before.

The truth is, regardless of what you go through, you start moving forward immediately. From the moment you experience loss, from the very first breath you take after the devastation, it happens regardless of your readiness and without your knowledge, because you don't have a choice.

Sit with that for a moment. You, right now, in your deepest and darkest grief, are moving forward already. There is a sense of peace in knowing you are already doing the hardest part. Even a moment filled with hopelessness is also filled with hope.

Here is another platitude I want to stick: "They'd want you to live this life . . . every moment of it." This platitude can be painful to hear, and often people say it without considering how it may make you feel. However, with years of experience behind me and after my seeing undeniable evidence in the lives of countless people, living is one of the best ways to find a positive path forward. I see living as an opportunity to honor what was lost and a way to lead by example for my children and the people I love who still walk this earth. By living I'm showing my children who their father was at his core and why he loved life. When people see you living your life they may assume you have moved on, but you will know the truth. Once you let go of the expectation to "move on," you can instead find joy in moving forward without the expectation to forget what came before.

MYTH 4

You Need to Be "Whole" Again

When we think of someone grieving, we—or your friends, family members, coworkers, etc.—may envision a person sitting in a corner, crying, being still and quiet for a defined amount of time until they eventually stand up whole and healed. That's not how grief works. Being "whole" is a myth. Once you lose a piece of yourself it is forever gone. It's not a question of filling a hole but rather using the void to evolve, grow, and change your perception of life's value.

You can love what was and love what is because love is not mutually exclusive and people are not replaceable; they do not leave behind holes to be filled over time. You will have to find your way through this darkness by reaching not to be *whole* again but to be *happy* again—to find peace with the circumstance at hand and start to establish a new normal. You may discover that your happiness has an ebb and flow, and on days when happiness appears it can disappear just as quickly. Life and grief have seasons; allow yourself the beauty of each season as it passes over you. It is all part of your taking steps forward.

MYTH 5

If You Aren't Crying, You Must Not Be Sad

I was cold and detached when I got the news of my late husband's crash. I don't think I cried for six months. To the outside eye, I was strong, aloof, and standoffish. I'm sure some judged my behavior and questioned my relationship with Mitch. What they didn't know is that when he died I also died . . . inside. The shock that covered my body was so extreme, most days I didn't feel a thing. It's hard to explain to anyone who has not experienced the power of that kind of shock, but I was a shell of a human walking around, going through the motions for nearly an entire year. Once I did feel the pain, in many ways I wanted the shock to come back.

For as many people who react in a similar way to me, there are countless others who react in the opposite way and every way in between. There is no correct reaction to grief. Your reaction will be based on your past and current life circumstances, your personality, and your body's ability to process stress, but never will it be based on the relationship you cherished with the person or people you lost. Don't let outside perceptions become your heart's reality. Your reaction is personal and should not be open for scrutiny.

MYTH 6

If You Talk About the Person You Lost, You Are Stuck

In 2015 I wrote a blog post about being a remarried widow who loved both my late husband, Mitch, and my current husband, Keith.[2] I've often joked that I didn't realize one blog post could break the Internet. The response to my words was incredible. I received so much support from people who felt validated in their emotions for perhaps the first time. I also faced so much anger from people who couldn't fathom that I could be remarried and still talk about Mitch, *and* have the audacity to say I loved them both. It has never seemed like a big deal to me. It's just my reality. I love what was and I love what is, and neither one is a replacement for the other; my heart is big and wide enough for both. I talk about Mitch all the time to his children, his friends, his parents, and even to myself. He was one of my favorite people, and he had an important impact on my life, so why would I just forget he ever existed? How is that healthy or true?

It's not. You don't forget the person you lost just because time passes or because you fall in love again. You don't replace a child that was lost with another child, so why would it be any different for the loss of a spouse? It's okay to talk about them if it feels right to you, and by remembering them, their light and life lives on. Don't let society tell you that you are stuck because you cherish memories and choose to say that loved one's name. I would argue that it is far healthier to tell the stories, laugh at the memories, and feel the love than to turn away and pretend they never existed. Your heart knows the truth, so don't hide your emotions to make others feel more comfortable. You aren't living for anyone but yourself, and that is the person you should honor as you take steps forward.

MYTH 7
Death Is the Hardest Part

The physical death of someone you love is painful and raw, but what many don't realize is that the physical death is just the beginning. The griever experiences countless losses after a death. My friend Christina Rasmussen talks about this kind of loss in her book *Second Firsts*.[3] Invisible losses are losses that come after death that are difficult to see and grieve and often hard to identify. These invisible losses are vast, and it would be impossible to list them all. Just a few examples are the loss of a planned future or the loss of support from the person who passed. The loss of security or self-worth. Watching your kids grow up without a parent; losing that person's financial contribution; missing the one person you told everything to; seeing your child play a sport for the first time with the realization that the other person who loved them as much as you do will never watch these moments with you—these invisible losses are real and painful, and unfortunately they continue for years to come. They are invisible to other people, who may believe you are doing well and moving forward. Frankly, your invisible losses are not their concern, and for the most part, they will not want to be bothered by your continued anguish.

These losses give you a new feeling that soon becomes familiar. I call it "duality"—when you find joy in the moment yet you feel the pain of your loss at the same time. Life after loss is full of duality, proving that emotions are complex and grief is anything but simple.

Duality and invisible losses are part of the process, but that does not mean you must feel alone. This is where a strong grief support system is vital. You need to surround yourself with positive energy and people who understand your pain but also will help you take steps forward with a growth mindset.

MYTH 8

The First Year Is the Hardest

Trust me when I say very few people will have patience for your grief beyond year one. That's not to say that the first year is the hardest, but people grow tired and just want you to *be okay already*. Speaking personally, year two was far harder for me than year one. I really felt the loss in year two physically, emotionally, and mentally. The shock had worn off, and I was fully aware of what I had endured. It became permanent and real as I accepted the reality I had not asked for. As I've carefully mentioned several times throughout this book—because it is so important—loss is individual, and each person has a unique process. Year one might be the worst for some and year ten for others. Don't judge your path, and don't worry what others think as you make your way forward.

MYTH 9

You Are an Inspiration

If I had a dollar for every time I've been told that I'm so strong or that I'm an inspiration, I'd be financially set for life. This seems to be the standard go-to response from onlookers viewing your tragedy from the outside. Your ability to function under the incredible circumstances you have been handed is inspiring to them, and for a brief time they may change their view on life and their status quo. I've never felt particularly strong or like an inspiration during my nearly eight years (at the writing of this book) since loss. Instead, I simply did what had to be done. I took care of my children, myself, and my personal priorities. I looked normal to the outside world, and my ability to get in phenomenal shape as well as start a business and a nonprofit seemed awe-inspiring to some, but for me it was just what I knew I had to do in the wake of a life-changing situation. People don't mean any harm by telling you that they feel inspired by your survival, but ultimately they don't realize the weight those words carry and that we place that weight squarely on our shoulders as an added responsibility. Don't hold the weight. Don't take it to heart and feel like you have to carry the world on your shoulders. You don't have to be anyone's inspiration, and you don't have to be strong. It's okay to recognize your ability to survive under the stress of loss, but it's never okay to think you have to be where you're not. You're allowed seasons of weakness as the world sees nothing but strength.

MYTH 10
You Will Get Unconditional Support

Not everyone in your life when you experience loss will be in your life after the loss. You will change in ways that many people will not like or respond to. I will never forget when someone told me that they wanted the old Michelle back. I laughed and said, "The old Michelle died when Mitch died. There is no getting her back, ever." People will leave your life for many reasons. Some can't deal with the pain, so they find it easier to walk away. Some don't like your growth or your inability to accept petty drama. Some just don't want to be bothered. You have to let them go, and let go of any negative energy surrounding their exit. You can't control how they feel, and you don't have the bandwidth to carry it with you. Let them go, and they may return to you some day. If they do, great. If they never return, it's a heartbreaking situation to have additional loss in your life, but unfortunately it's very real. Please remember, it's most likely not about you. You can't own their feelings; don't even try.

You will also find yourself judged for your many choices after your loss. I always found it curious that nobody seemed to care about my life with Mitch before he died, but after, I felt as if I were living in a glass house of grief.[4] Suddenly everyone cared about my life and every move I was making. One day, long after my loss, I read *The Four Agreements* by Don Miguel Ruiz and took a new viewpoint on the glass house I was living in. I came to the realization that it wasn't about me and I shouldn't take the judgment of other people personally or make assumptions about what they were thinking. If you haven't read *The Four Agreements,* I can't recommend it enough. It will alter how you see life after loss. It helped me grow experientially and let go of other people's perceptions.

The Gifts of Grief: Post-Traumatic Growth

As you very well know at this moment, grief is ongoing. Your loss has evolved from a single moment into a constant barrage of losses that you feel for weeks, months, years. I want you to move through this pain, in it, and with it. I want you to feel it as it moves and shifts because it will forever change the course of your life. I want you to take even the smallest steps each day to process your loss, absorb it into who you are becoming, and allow it to change you for the better. Let me say it again because it is so important: *You can use this pain to change for the better.* In fact, this is the enormous gift of grief; it propels you toward change.

Interestingly enough, in the mid-1990s, the term "post-traumatic growth" was coined by psychologists Richard G. Tedeschi and Lawrence G. Calhoun at the University of North Carolina, and their study shed light on what many grieving people feel.[5] PTG is basically the positive change experienced after life-altering circumstances, such as trauma or crisis. The idea is that humans can be changed, often for the better, after emerging from struggle. PTG can have an effect on everything from the opportunities perceived by the person affected to how relationships are handled and often results in a much greater appreciation for life. Shawn Achor, a Harvard psychologist, talks about this phenomenon in his book *The Happiness Advantage,* and as soon as I read the words "post-traumatic growth," I knew it was giving scientific backing to something I'd recognized in the grief world for a very long time. You can actually become a better version of yourself after trauma, and that fact alone can give you hope for a better future.

Even if you are experiencing PTG at this very moment, you may feel damaged and anything but hopeful. But I can tell you that grief does not make you a damaged person. It enlightens you if you allow it to. Loss teaches us to appreciate the moment, to love what matters, that life is less about stuff and more about experiences and memories. Loss teaches us that we have a finite amount of time to do all those things we've dreamed of doing. We love more deeply and give more freely. Loss is perhaps the greatest teacher available to humankind, and as the survivor of loss, you too are now enlightened with the gifts of grief. While I wouldn't wish my pain on my worst enemy, I would wish my perspective of life on the entire world. If every human walking this planet had this perspective, we'd live in a kinder, gentler, and—I would argue—more fulfilled world.

Our darkest moments offer many of the greatest growth opportunities. Sometimes clarity, intuition, and perspective collide, and we are given the chance to either charge forward boldly or gently slip back. We stand at the fork in the road, looking at all the signs laid out before us, and we decide whether we will find the strength and inner fortitude to maneuver the rough terrain of the bumpy unknown. If you have said good-bye to the person you never thought you could live without and you are here reading my words right now, I know you are powerful and limitless. You have lived with the worst, and you are thereby capable of doing just about anything you dream possible. I ask you, as you stand at this fork in your road, to choose fitness as part of your forward path. With fitness as your ally on this journey, you will be able to face the hard days with more confidence, strength, and inner peace.

I know what you are thinking: *Michelle, I can hardly get out of bed. I'm devastated, exhausted, and just trying to survive. I don't think I can add fitness to my life right now. Where would I start? What would I do? Will it really help me?*

Perhaps knowing more about the connection between exercise and its effects on your brain, body, and mood might help motivate you. Let's explore the science behind what fitness does for your physical, mental, and emotional states. The facts don't lie, and I guarantee that by the time you finish the next chapter, you'll want to start moving.

CHAPTER 2

Your Grief on Endorphins

When I started writing about the importance of fitness as a grief-coping tool I took some serious heat for my claims. I will never forget an angry email I received from a woman who thought my fitness coping strategy was making light of a serious situation. Her exact words were "Do you really think me walking on a treadmill is going to make me okay?"

Let me be clear: I've never once said that fitness will "fix" or "take away" grief. Sadly, there is no way to ever take away your pain. Remember those myths I mentioned in the previous chapter? Your grief will forever be a part of who you are, and rather than looking for ways to "fix" it, I'd prefer to help you process and cope with it in a healthy, productive, and life-affirming manner. Ironically, the woman emailed me back about a year later and apologized for her outburst; she admitted she just hadn't been ready to hear the information I had been trying to give her. She told me that she started a walking program shortly after our exchange, and it did indeed help her cope with her loss.

Prescribing Exercise

It's not exactly newsworthy that fitness can be a powerful and life-changing tool, yet it's not often mentioned by grief counselors, doctors, or support groups. It's not widely accepted as a go-to method of therapy, but it's my hope that through this book and further education on its clear and powerful benefits, fitness will become one of the first forms of therapy prescribed by health professionals, discussed by grief groups, covered in grief pamphlets, and more widely talked about in grief books.

Doctors and therapists alike have been studying exercise for years, and there is more than enough concrete evidence to prove that exercise changes your brain, your mood, and your overall feelings about life. Despite the evidence, it's still an afterthought by many health professionals. We've become a nation of quick fixes and prescription pills. It's often faster and easier for a doctor to give you a pill than encourage you to be an advocate for your own healthy healing. Your body is an amazing machine full of healing properties. In most cases, your body already has everything it needs to move you in a positive direction and gain new strength. In fact, if the pharmaceutical industry could bottle the power of fitness and harness it in pill form, it would be arguably the most widely prescribed medicine in history.

In thinking about her email again, though, I would argue that, yes, walking on a treadmill *is* going to make you, in a way, better. And there are some powerful scientific studies to back up this claim.

The Fitness Prescription

My general physician gave me some sage advice when I visited her about eight months after my loss. I remember telling her that I felt gray, cloudy, and lost. It is called "widow brain," "grief brain," and "brain fog," but regardless of the name, the outcome is the same: it's hard to think, to process information, and to make sense of the small things. This fog can be chalked up to stress, shock, anxiety, and overwhelming life circumstances. The grayness was very real and frustrating. Another invisible loss seemed to be stealing my ability to function at a level I was accustomed to.

This particular doctor had seen my life at all stages. She was with me before I had children and after. She'd seen me overweight and sedentary, active and healthy. She knew the toll my loss had taken on me, but she also knew the deep fortitude I'd call upon to work through the loss. Still, I felt as if I needed assistance to help get beyond the shock my body was still experiencing all those months later.

Often we fall back on taking a pill and hoping the pharmaceutical companies have figured out a fix so we don't have to. Don't get me wrong; there are very real conditions that require medication. But prescriptions for widows are often antidepressants, antianxiety medications, and pain pills. While you may need one of these things at some point in your journey, my goal in writing this book is to give you other options. In many cases, your body can help itself if you do what it needs you to do.

My brain fog was actually a sign that my body was still processing grief. The body is an incredibly intricate and powerful multisystem problem solver. It is designed to protect us from trauma, to help us survive. The fog was a shield from painful memories; it was my body trying to help me. As I sat in my doctor's office and told her that perhaps I needed an antidepressant, she asked, "Michelle, do you have moments of the day when you don't feel the fog?" My response was immediate and honest: "Yes, but only after I exercise." She wrote a few notes on her paper and then asked another question. "Do you find any exercise better than another to help?" Again, I replied without thinking: "Yes, it's always better after I run." She took a few more notes and then looked up from her paper and said something that would forever shape my world: "Michelle, there is nothing better I can give you in this office than what you do for yourself in that gym every day. Endorphins are the best antidepressant on the market, and they are completely free!"

What's Going On in There?

There is irrefutable evidence that movement makes us not only healthier but happier too. More studies are being conducted in this field all the time, and the mounting support is undeniable. When we move our bodies, our brains retain information better and become less cloudy, we have more energy, and we feel more alive. With movement, we are better able to adapt, grow, and evolve, which is critical when dealing with any type of grief. *Adapting* to new circumstances, challenges, and a new normal—which seems to happen daily in a post-loss world—can be better faced when movement is applied. *Growing* into a new life, a new role, with a new future requires us to adapt while also *evolving* and being flexible enough to handle new obstacles.

One of my favorite books on the subject of exercise for the brain and the brain's connection to the body is John J. Ratey's *Spark*. In this fantastic book, Dr. Ratey writes, "Neuroscientists have just begun studying exercise's impact within brain cells—at the genes themselves. Even there, in the roots of our biology, they've found signs of the body's influence on the mind. It turns out that moving our muscles produces proteins that travel through the bloodstream and into the brain, where they play pivotal roles in the mechanisms of our highest thought processes. They bear names such as insulin-like growth factor (IGF-1) and vascular endothelial growth factor (VEGF), and they provide an unprecedented view of the mind–body connection."[1] What Dr. Ratey and researchers like him are finding is that a connection is made between the mental and physical when we exercise, and this connection is vital to our mental health.

We need to move and we know it! Our bodies are hardwired to crave physical output, and when we give the body what it needs it rewards us with a host of benefits. These are not just placebo effects—exercise changes the body at a cellular level. In this chapter I'm going to give you a layperson's breakdown of what happens in your body as a direct result of exercise so you can understand this process a little more. I promise to make it quick! Remember, I'm not a doctor or a scientist, but, lucky for us, the science of brain changes through exercise is becoming a widely studied field.

When you exercise or move your body there are a few different things going on I want to talk about. Movement is essentially a "stress" on your body, and when we stress our bodies they become stronger. Your brain recognizes these movements as either fight or flight situations. In order for your body to protect itself, chemical reactions release proteins. One chemical reaction in particular helps you to better deal with stress by producing proteins called BDNF (brain derived neurotrophic factor). These BDNF proteins have been shown to help with fighting anxiety and depression, along with increasing your mental ability. While all this is going on in the brain, it is also manufacturing endorphins, which help to minimize stress. These endorphins act as analgesics, meaning they have the ability to diminish your perception of pain. The powerful combinations of BDNF and endorphins are the reason you feel good when you exercise and are said to have the same addictive properties as drugs such as heroine, morphine, and nicotine. We could consider endorphins natural drugs because they activate receptors in the brain that minimize discomfort and can bring on feelings of euphoria and well-being. John Ratey refers to them as "Miracle-Gro for the brain." He goes on to say, "Exercise is the single most powerful tool you have to optimize your brain function."[2] Research from Dr. Ratey and many others has found that not only does exercise make you feel better, but it improves brain function as well, which can feel even more critical when you're facing traumatic and stressful life events.

While that is a simplistic view of what is going on all over your body, it gives you enough information to understand that movement—truly of any kind—is beneficial for your entire system and should be used daily to improve all areas of your life.

Convinced? Let me follow the science up with a few personal stories of how exercise brought about positive change after major life difficulties. I think this will help you see the power of exercise and brain science in action.

The Transformative Power of Exercise

Over the years since I created One Fit Widow, I've heard countless stories from grieving people who have had the same life-affirming relationship with exercise as I have. I'd love to share just a few of their stories with you before you begin this program yourself.

I'm not so focused on the external transformation as I am on the internal transformation, but it seems they parallel each other. I'll start with the present: I am in training for my first full Ironman in Chattanooga. . . . I completed my first half Ironman last year and have been working hard to even think this insane goal was something I could attain. Now I know it *is*.

My "why" I'm doing this came through a series of events that started on October 27, 2005, when we put our eighteen-month-old daughter, Hannah, to bed and she never woke up. This changed the course of our lives forever. It took me eight long years (of doing things that did not help) to figure out that running, biking, and swimming are where Hannah comes to meet me. Those are my sacred spaces. But sometimes the challenges of grief and sorrow can outweigh the desire to train. On the days my body feels like my bones are made of stone, I use all the physical, mental, and emotional strength I have to try to equate the physical pain to the emotional pain of the deepest sorrow. Those are the times my body grows strong. Grief has a persistent course, and I've learned that I can work *with* this persistent course instead of against it. When I look back to when I started my exercise as a form of grief work in 2013, my confidence began to grow. My ability to function in a world without my living daughter became about finding moments out on the trails with her. The wind that would blow my hair was filled with her. The heart-shaped leaf with the outline of the sun silhouetted underwater, on a frigid cold morning lake swim in Michigan, was her way of cheering me on. I want my two living children to learn that life is hard. Life is not fair. Life is struggle. And life is unbelievably beautiful in all its tragedy. Everything I do now is to honor Hannah's legacy and teach my other two kids about how to stand up when you get knocked down.

As for the physical aspect, in the past four years, I dropped about 50 to 60 pounds. The intense training coming this summer

will take more off, just because of the nature of Ironman training. But the physical part is the last part of the puzzle for me. I'm
grateful to be able to breath, to run and chase my kids, to climb
the sand dunes with them and ride roller coasters. I have energy
and I want to live, really live and be alive. Death has a way of
opening up Life!

—*Tracy Mitchell*

The first five months after Matt passed I was lost in a very thick
fog. Stuck in a perpetual state of numbness where I somehow
made it through everyday but only on autopilot. The autopilot
consisted mostly of ignoring the fact that I was a thirty-one-
year-old widow that started my dream job just two weeks after
my husband died. Somehow I was learning this new job while
being completely detached to the moving world around me. I
would go to work, do my best, and then cry the second I left
the building and my entire drive home. At home one of my
parents would arrive shortly to stay the night with me. I would
take an over-the-counter sleeping pill around 9 so I'd be in
bed by 9:30 and asleep at 10. This cycle continued for five
months. What happened around five months was that my sister forced—or we will say encouraged—me to sign up for the
Portland Shamrock 5K. She had been running for many years
now, and I had never run a day in my life. I thought this was
dumb, but it always looked like she had fun at racing events.
When race day came I was nervous because I hadn't really
trained. In a strange way I was also excited about all the positive
energy around me. It was contagious! We started the race, and
not shortly into it I walked, then jogged a little, walked more,

jogged a little, and basically walked the rest. The 5K took me fifty-five minutes to complete, but I did it. It was after that race I decided I needed to maybe put more effort into this running thing, as I clearly couldn't wing it. Plus, these crazy people who loved running seemed so ecstatic about life and I wanted that. So I started going with my sister every Thursday to a local run group. My family was encouraging of this, as it got me out and socializing with people. I'd do a mile out and then a mile back. As the weeks and months went by, I got faster, and my two miles turned into the full three. It was just eight months into my running adventure that I spontaneously signed up for a 12K with the help of my sister. I thought I'd die right there on the course and likely see my dead husband standing over me laughing and calling me a fool. He was funny like that. But I didn't die. I pushed through that course and completed the seven miles in 1:32:58, averaging a 12'14-minute mile. This was a major accomplishment for me. I pushed myself beyond what I thought I could do. Running was therapy for me. Hate and sadness poured out of me with every drop of sweat. I hated that my husband made me a widow at thirty-one. However, it was sweating out the sadness and all the emotions that accompany grief that I believe helped me heal and quicker than if I hadn't found running. Running brought me to a new social group in a time when I could have easily isolated myself. I also began to lose weight and that boosted my confidence. These positive changes I received in my life from just running were priceless. I truly feel if running hadn't found me I would be in a deep dark depression. Running saved me when I couldn't see through the fog of being a widow.

—*Rachelle Nunes*

In 2010, my husband was killed in a car accident on his way home from work at the age of thirty-two. He was four miles from home. My oldest son was two at the time and I was four and a half months pregnant with my second son. I was a runner and continued to run throughout my pregnancy, with my doctor's approval. I was determined not to take medication since I was pregnant after my husband died. Exercise was the only thing that would make me feel better. I craved it. After my son was born, I immediately started back as soon as I got my doctor's approval. In 2011, a tornado hit my house while I was home with my children. My youngest was seven weeks old. The damage done to my home was enough that we had to move out for two months for repairs. Even during that time, I continued to exercise. I couldn't have made it without having that release. In 2013, I trained and ran my first half marathon. I cried when I crossed the finish line. I knew my late husband would have been so proud of me. To this day, I continue to exercise several times a week. I've never had to take medication for depression, and I attribute that to exercising. It's my medicine and my breath of fresh air. I remarried in November 2016 to a wonderful man that loves me and my boys. I gained a daughter through that as well. I went through some rough times, but I never got in a deep state of depression. I attribute that to exercise and prayer!

—*Angela West*

You can find more stories for inspiration at the Healthy Healing online portal.

A Cultural Problem

Our sedentary lifestyle and conditioning start at a very early age with a de-emphasis on movement. Especially now that I have my own young kids, I find it disheartening how we try to teach children life skills, such as mathematical equations, important historical dates, and valuable literature, all while asking them to sit in school as still as possible. I see this as an overarching issue with education (I will save that for a later book); we spend years developing what's in their heads while ignoring their bodies and other key development factors, such as vital 3-D learning. It's as if we've disconnected their brains from their little bodies because somehow we believe the two are mutually exclusive. This is a terrible mistake, as our bodies and brains work in conjunction, not separately, and any movement will only benefit all aspects of the education process. An even bigger issue is that when we deprioritize exercise for young people, the habit of non-movement carries into their adulthood, and we end up with an entire population who doesn't make exercise the priority it should be. It's typically the first thing to suffer when our lives get the hardest.

On the flip side, when we are allowed to move throughout the day, we are more focused and think more critically. This is true, of course, for both children and adults and is the reason so many large companies are adapting wellness programs and putting fitness centers in their corporate offices. Some of the most productive and "happiest" companies in the world, such as Virgin Atlantic, Google, and Mindvalley, have largely adapted a full-body approach, incorporating not only fitness but mindfulness via meditation. As John J. Ratey so eloquently discusses in his book *Spark,* "We must bring the head and the body back together, not only for better learning but the creation of happier, more energetic, overall more productive human beings."[3]

Movement and Disease

Now that we understand the scientific connection between exercise and our brains and bodies, we can make the additional link between lack of movement and depression, anxiety, and PTSD, often experienced by people who are grieving.

DEPRESSION

According to the World Health Organization, at least 300 million people of all ages suffer from depression worldwide, and it is the leading cause of disability.[4] The Centers for Disease Control and Prevention report that the United States is among the countries most deeply affected by depression.[5] These staggering numbers are affecting not only many people's abilities to have happy and fulfilled lives, but depression costs in "treatment, disability, and lost productivity are comparable to the dollars spent on heart disease," according to Dr. Linn Goldberg, author of the book *The Healing Power of Exercise*.[6] Depression is crippling large parts of our society and we are in desperate need of ways to combat this growing epidemic.

Depression is much more serious than just feeling sad or down for a few days. Depression creates accompanying negative feelings that stay with you most of the time and can leave you feeling like you've lost all interest and pleasure in life. Often with depression it can become difficult to think clearly or sleep well, and it can sometimes lead to feelings of suicide and intense guilt.

So what causes depression and how can you avoid being one of the thousands of grievers who experience its symptoms? According to Harvard Health, it's much more complicated than most people realize. "It's often said that depression results from a chemical imbalance, but that figure of speech does not capture how complex the disease is.

Benefits of Regular Exercise

Some of the known benefits of regular exercise include

- Potentially increased life span

- More energy

- Better mood

- Better sleep

- Improved self-confidence and self-esteem

- Sharper thinking and mental clarity

- Greater personal resilience

- Reduced risk of numerous health issues, such as heart disease, stroke, certain forms of cancer, high blood pressure, diabetes (both prevention and treatment), high cholesterol and triglyceride levels, and glaucoma

- Fat burning and muscle building

- Bone strengthening

- Reduced stress, anxiety, and symptoms of depression

Research suggests that depression doesn't spring from simply having too much or too little of certain brain chemicals. Rather, depression has many possible causes, including faulty mood regulation by the brain, genetic vulnerability, stress life events, medications, and medical problems."[7]

Despite the fact that we don't yet know exactly what affects our propensity for depression, we are figuring out ways to deal with its negative effects. According to *Psychology Today,* over twenty-five case studies confirm that exercise helps prevent depression. "Professors from the University of Toronto have compiled and analyzed over twenty-six years' worth of scientific research, which concludes that even moderate levels of physical activity—like walking for twenty to thirty minutes a day—can ward off depression in people of all ages. University of Toronto PhD candidate George Mammen coauthored a review of twenty-five different research articles, which show that moderate exercise can prevent episodes of depression in the long term. The compilation of research is published in the October issue of the *American Journal of Preventive Medicine.*"[8]

ANXIETY AND PTSD

Many of us know what anxiety feels like: heart beating out of your chest, trouble breathing, lightheadedness, shaking hands or restless legs, and sometimes extreme panic. *Merriam-Webster* describes anxiety as "a fear or nervousness about what might happen" and "an abnormal and overwhelming sense of apprehension and fear often marked by physical signs (such as tension, sweating, and increased pulse rate), by doubt concerning the reality and nature of the threat, and by self-doubt about one's capacity to cope with it."[9] Grief and anxiety go hand in hand in many cases. When you have lived through traumatic circumstances your body processes situations differently than it did before. If you get better at identifying anxiety when it comes up, you can combat it with useful techniques, like exercise, meditation, solid nutrition, and deep breathing.

According to the Mayo Clinic, "post-traumatic stress disorder (PTSD) is a mental health condition that's triggered by a terrifying event—either experiencing it or witnessing it. Symptoms may include flashbacks, nightmares, and severe anxiety, as well as uncontrollable thoughts about the event."[10] I first realized that I might have

Seeking Help for Depression

I can't stress enough how important it is to talk with your doctor if you are experiencing any of the emotions associated with depression. Many of these feelings are a part of the grief process so you may not be clinically depressed, but that is for your doctor and you to figure out. Physicians do feel that exercise can be used effectively to treat mild to moderate forms of depression, so also talk with your doctor about incorporating fitness and let them advise you on the best path forward.

PTSD shortly after my late husband's crash. Once the shock wore off, I'd find myself having anxiety over the well-being of the people closest in my life. I'd begin to feel anxiety when I didn't receive a return phone call or text from someone or when I watched the news. I made some life adjustments, continued my exercise routine, and managed the anxiety without medication. About two years after my loss I was driving on the same freeway that had been stopped with traffic the day of his crash, and I looked across the street and saw a very bad accident. In that moment my body absolutely came apart. I began to sweat, feel intense anxiety, and have trouble breathing. Additional instances over the next year convinced me to talk with my doctor and counselor, who confirmed that I may have a mild form of PTSD. I remember hearing "PTSD" and feeling so damaged. However, I learned, once again, that fitness could play a major role in helping me regulate my anxiety and PTSD symptoms. According to Matthew Tull, PhD, "Several studies have looked at the effect of a regular exercise program on PTSD symptoms. In one study of adolescents with PTSD, it was found that those who took part in an aerobic exercise program for forty minutes, three times per week, for a total of eight weeks, experienced a reduction in PTSD symptoms, anxiety, and depression. In another study of adults with PTSD, a twelve-session aerobic exercise program was found to also lead to a decrease in PTSD symptoms, depression, and anxiety after the program ended."[11]

Exercise for Sleep and Mental Clarity

The intense fog in the brain often associated with grief can be frustrating to overcome. To help diminish brain fog, ensure you get a good night's sleep. A lot of positive things happen in your brain and your body when you sleep. Your blood pressure plummets, the extra mental "trash" you accumulate during the day gets cleared out, and of course your body creates important growth hormones. However, sleep can be hard to come by when you are experiencing life-altering grief. What helps you get the sleep you need? You guessed it: exercise.

Besides the obvious physical exhaustion that accompanies a solid training program, regular exercise can trigger an increase in body temperature, followed by a postexercise drop in temperature, both of which promote sleep later. Another benefit is that the exerciser may see a reduction in insomnia, thanks to a decrease in anxiety and depressive symptoms.[12] When exercise and good sleep are used together, you will be able to tackle grief more effectively.

The Life-Saving Power of Exercise

I only realized the true power of fitness after I experienced devastating loss. I accidentally fell into a therapy that literally saved my life. Nobody told me to go train in my early days after loss. Nobody encouraged me to work out for my mental health. In fact, many people couldn't believe that I was taking the time for a run or an hour at the gym. They thought I was focusing on something unimportant and vain at a time when I should have been weeping on the floor. They didn't realize how important that hour of time was to my overall life and grief management. They didn't realize that the only way I survived my loss in those first few months was to sweat it out. I knew how important it was right away, and with each passing workout I realized more and more that I needed to spend the rest of my life making sure every person who grieves knows it too.

The wonderful thing about adding in an exercise program for better overall mental health is that there are no negative side effects. You can take a ten-minute daily walk and reap the rewards both physically and mentally, and see the results immediately in your sleep, your energy levels, and your resilience. More often than not, your greatest challenge is overcoming the obstacles to get started.

So there you have it: the facts. In the next chapters I'm going to introduce you to the two main components of the twelve-week Healthy Healing program: exercise and nutrition. It's important that you understand the basics before you hit the ground (literally) running.

CHAPTER 3

Exercise

I get how hard it is to start exercising, especially when you're experiencing life-altering grief. Some days simply getting out of bed may feel like a major success. I want you always to honor and celebrate the baby steps you take each day, but I also want you to understand that the days when you least want to take those steps are the very days you need them the most. The days when you are deep in despair and questioning a life beyond the person you lost are the days when you should trust your body's ability to help you. I've often found that when I have to fight my inner demons and really talk myself into movement, I have the best workout and really connect to my own healing power after I'm done.

But where do you begin? As a woman who has experienced the power of fitness for the grieving soul, I'd love to tell you to dive right into an intense exercise routine, to go hard, sweat until you cry, and never give up. But as a fitness coach and, more importantly, a woman who has been overweight, tired, and out of shape, I recognize the importance of baby steps in all aspects of life and especially in your quest for fitness. Your readiness to use exercise as a grief-coping mechanism will ultimately come down to your current fitness level and your personality type. You may want to jump in right away or you may get overwhelmed by the concept of change. Human beings tend to take the path of least resistance, and that is why a quick change rarely translates into a long-term change. Making sweeping changes may be easy for a few days or even a few weeks, but most people eventually fall back into old habits, and suddenly the new ways seem like too much work to sustain. You will be much better off starting with a small set of changes and enlarging that set over time. This helps remap the brain and bring about lasting change.

In this chapter you will take the most important baby steps and choose your first forms of exercise. Often the kind of movement that serves you well will depend on the waves of grief you are currently experiencing. Whatever forms you pick, remember that gradual

The Duality of Grief

As you exercise, the movement will push you forward. The pain will wash over your tired body, helping to give a deep strength to your exhausted soul. By pushing your body, you are expanding your senses, experiencing a physical release that is cathartic beyond anything I can explain with simple words. Exercise may be the first time you feel the duality that is grief—the happiness of personal accomplishment coupled with the sadness of doing it *without them*. This duality will be your new companion and will accompany you for the rest of your days. Nearly all happy moments will have a touch of pain, though the pain will eventually no longer debilitate you. The duality will remind you of life's preciousness and your limited time to do all the things you dream of doing. Fitness will give rise to those dreams and power to your altered future.

progress is best. Your body needs baby steps, now more than ever, and any significant changes can lead quickly to injury, fatigue, or burnout, which will force you to quit. Go slowly, add a little more activity day by day, and remember that movement creates change. That's the key to this book. I want you to work toward being not only physically fit but mentally and emotionally fit as well. Healthy healing is not just about your body; it's about your life.

The next words I'm going to say to you are imperative, and I want you to write them someplace and refer to them often:

Whatever you do, don't get overwhelmed,
and whatever you do, don't quit!

This program may seem daunting and scary, but don't quit before you even start. I'll take it slow and help make fitness easy for you in the pages ahead. You'll be able to figure out what you need and how to make it not only a part of your day but a part of your life. In part two of this book I outline a twelve-week workout and life-restructuring program, but please understand, my way is not the only way. There is no right or wrong workout, and there is no foolproof program. Only consistency, persistence, and patience will lead you to success.

The best way to combat the urge to quit is to find a form of exercise that you love and do what works for you in the moment. The important thing is not how you move but rather that you do indeed move—flooding your brain with endorphins and taking those daily steps in a forward direction.

It is also important that you keep your choices limited and abide by the twenty-second rule: it should take you only twenty seconds to get ready for your workout. At whatever time of the day you've decided to work out, figure out ahead of time what form of exercise you are going to do that day, and ready your clothing or gym bag beforehand, so you avoid the temptation to be overwhelmed when the time comes. Limit your choices so you cannot fall prey to mental pitfalls.

Now I'm going to walk you through several forms of exercise, explaining the benefits of each and why some are particularly therapeutic during the grieving process. Let's start nice and easy because sometimes it only takes a little change to make a big impact.

Walking

Walking is one of my favorite activities. I try to take my dogs on at least a two-mile walk daily, regardless of what else I've done in the gym. Walking clears my head, fills my heart, and expands my soul. I leave the electronics at home and embrace the quiet, or sometimes I take my favorite audiobook or podcast and use the time to work on my personal growth. More often than not, I choose the quiet and embrace my inner voice.

This can be a very scary concept to someone who is grieving. It may be difficult to be alone, to think and go into yourself, but it is a critical step in your health and the way you process your grief. With even just a ten- to twenty-minute walk, preferably in nature, you will change the chemical reactions within your brain. Remember the "grief brain" and the BDNF protein I explained earlier? Walking is fantastic for your grief brain, and you may find a window of time after your walk when you can make important decisions, take care of paperwork, and even smile at friends or family before the intensity of the pain returns. Your brain and body love walking, and in my experience, so does your heart. After years of training and fitness, walking is no longer what I do exclusively for fitness, but it is a critical part of my emotional health and well-being. It is the easiest and most efficient way just to get started. No special equipment needed, no expensive gym membership, just a nice walk out your front door to move you forward.

If you are new to exercise, start with a simple walk. Aim small in the beginning and make it so easy that you can't talk yourself out of it. Tell yourself that you will walk—again, preferably outside (nature is important for many reasons I will soon explain)—for just ten minutes on day one. We can all make time for a ten-minute walk. With this baby-step goal, you are setting yourself up for success. If you get outside, walk for ten minutes, and find that you don't want to quit, then just keep on going. It certainly won't hurt to go farther, but just promise yourself every part of that full ten minutes. Each day add one more minute to your walk, and pay careful attention to how you feel before, during, and after your walk. While you walk, focus on breathing deeply. If possible, leave all electronics at home and disconnect from the noise and clutter of life. Enjoy the fresh air while taking as many cleansing breaths as possible. Continue this pattern and notice your strength compound by the day.

Once you are addicted to how it makes you feel, keep going. Work your way up to newer and stronger forms of exercise, such as running.

Running / Jogging

Running was my preferred form of therapy in my first year after loss. I needed to run that first year because the cardiovascular endorphins helped me feel unstoppable. Just like walking, running is a metaphor for life. You look forward, you put one foot in front of the other, and you pound the pavement and forget the world. I believe it to be one of the most powerful ways to cope with grief.

Running elicits a flood of endorphins to the brain, and because it can be intense, the positive effects of the endorphins are felt more quickly and with more force—a "runner's high"—and the compelling benefits are strongly associated with mood elevation and happiness.

You may have to work your body up to running. Please always remember the importance of gradual progress, but once you've conditioned yourself to run or jog, you may never want to stop. It's a euphoric feeling, and you may find yourself drowning in tears that had been bottled up and needed to be shed. Running can bring it all forward. I remember training for the San Diego marathon after Mitch passed. I'd run outside in my neighborhood, and the long runs would cause the tears to fall fast and furious as my body was flooded with every possible emotion, from pain to anger to uncontrollable sadness to, eventually, pride. There was a particular gratification in my pushing forward and surviving despite the tragic cards I'd been dealt. It was not fair, but I was not done.

Once you master running, you can increase your intensity until you begin to sprint. Sprinting takes conditioning, but once you start it will expand the therapy of running tenfold. You leave it all there on the pavement, and your body experiences a unique connection to your mind's power. When you run that hard and that fast you start to believe the words "I am unstoppable."

If you want to move toward sprinting, I again strongly suggest you gradually condition your body for it. A good way to begin is to sprint for thirty to forty-five seconds, and after each burst allow your body to recover as you walk for thirty to forty-five seconds. Repeat the process for ten to twenty repetitions, and work your way up with each workout.

This type of interval training has a name—high-intensity interval training, or HIIT—and it is particularly effective in helping the body feel better as well as being key to neurogenesis, or the development of new brain neurons (more on this later in the book too).

Swimming

With swimming, you may discover a wave of peace unique to the flow, weightlessness, and stillness of the water. The body largely consists of water, and water is literally and symbolically a source of life. Surrounding yourself in its power can work wonders. Psychologists have long recognized the meditative and healing qualities of water through swimming. Even the sound of a lapping pool or a running river can produce a measurable effect on the body. Wave patterns in the brain alter in a way very similar to when we meditate or relax. Swimming can connect us powerfully to our bodies, and many people say it reminds them of being in the womb or of our evolutionarily past.

Another great benefit of swimming is that it's gentle on your body. If you have joint issues, back problems, mobility limitations, or extra fat to lose, walking or running can be difficult. Swimming is an effective alternative. You can start with a walking program in the water, or you can add in light swimming and water resistance training. Anything you can do on land you can do in the water and with added resistance. You will not only receive the same benefits of land exercise, both physically and emotionally, but also save your body the wear and tear sometimes associated with traditional training. For anyone struggling to start, getting in the pool can be a wonderful way to move your body as well as enjoy exercise for perhaps the first time.

If you can find the right place to swim, it can be a year-round exercise option that will be excellent for your mind, body, and soul. Your new swimming routine will help keep your heart working properly, improve lung function, take stress off your body, and help you maintain a healthy weight. You will gain endurance, strengthen those muscles, and improve your overall cardiovascular health. Finally, because swimming offers a total body workout, you won't have to worry about what part of your body you're missing. As you become stronger, you can take on more challenging workouts and trade off weightlessness in the water for the release of lifting weights.

A great way to get started swimming is to try simple strokes, like the breaststroke or backstroke, and gradually increase the amount of laps you do at one time. Start with one lap (down and back) and then allow your heart rate to recover and your body to rest before you add another lap. Keep building each time you enter the pool. Once you find yourself more conditioned, you can start with a five-minute warm-up, attempting not to stop, and work on lengthening and stretching out the strokes. Then attempt six laps with a twenty- to thirty-second rest in between each. Progress from there by gradually adding laps.

As a side note, you may find the backstroke to be particularly beneficial, as your ears are submerged under the water and you experience the added quiet that comes from being surrounded by stillness.

Resistance Training

You may find that as you move through your grief, you need to utilize different kinds of exercise therapy. What works for you during the first few months of your grief and fitness journey might not work in later months. What once was your saving grace may become like a chore, so you have to be willing to evolve with your routine. Just like life, you are a fluid being and your needs change with your season, emotions, and current life circumstance.

Depending on where you are in your grief journey, resistance training can be an incredibly rewarding and life-altering experience. As a fitness coach, I believe that resistance training is one of the most

A Strong Silhouette, Not a Bulky Body

For the ladies reading this book, I want to dispel the notion that resistance training will make you bulky. This is an age-old myth that is not founded in fact. The truth is, building muscle is a difficult and time-consuming process. Women do not have the high levels of testosterone in their bodies required to get "big," and lifting weights—resistance training—when combined with the right foods, will ultimately make you smaller. Muscles are dense and compact, and they create long lines, so when you start to shed fat, you become longer and leaner too. Don't be scared to pick up the weights for your best body and your best stress relief.

effective ways to change your body. It reduces your chances of osteoporosis by increasing bone density, fights depression, lowers your risk of diabetes, supports heart health, helps overall balance, and improves mental strength. By adding lean muscle mass, you also increase your resting metabolism, so you end up burning more fat, even while at rest. As you shed fat and add lean muscle, you may not see the scale change dramatically, but you will notice your body becoming stronger, leaner, and faster as it starts to operate at its most effective level.

Obviously I can speak to the health benefits of nearly any form of exercise, but as a grieving mother, I can tell you that resistance training has a distinct place in the grief journey. Grief is ripe with anger, and we experience it at various times during our journey. We all have moments when we ask "Why me?" and "Why them?" I've been angry more times than I care to admit. Even years later, I still have waves of anger. When the anger gets so intense you feel like you need to hit something or scream at the top of your lungs, resistance training can provide a safe, healthy outlet. When you push and resist the weight, you can harness your pain and use it for the betterment of your mind, body, and spirit. The anger is going to come—it is an inevitable part of the journey—so why not face it while gaining inner and outer strength? You may even find that it becomes addictive and fun. I was always the girl who didn't like lifting heavy weights because I wanted to stay skinny, but later I realized that lifting weights has nothing to do with my size, and strong beats skinny any day!

Kickboxing / Boxing

Why kickboxing or boxing? Because sometimes you just need to hit something really hard again and again.

As I said before, anger is a very real part of grief, and you need a positive outlet for that anger. Let's not pretend that it doesn't exist; let's instead figure out how anger can benefit us physically and emotionally. Everything I just said about weight lifting applies to activities like kickboxing and boxing. This form of exercise allows you to move your anger in a positive direction and physically break through the pain. You may even find you yell or scream as you hit the bag, and that's okay. You are releasing an energy your body needs to work through, and you are getting stronger in the process. Not to mention that kickboxing provides an intense cardio workout, just like running gives you that flood of cleansing endorphins.

Kickboxing and boxing are also very effective at helping build confidence as well as additional positive coping mechanisms. Kickboxing is founded in traditional martial arts, which prepare your warrior mind and spirit. It can help improve decision making and calm anxiety. When we grieve, on top of the basic fear that comes with the loss

Box Breathing

Kickboxing helps you learn proper breathing techniques, and this is important because in times of great stress we often forget to breathe deeply. We may instead breathe in irregular patterns, which is not good for your body and often contributes to anxiety or stress. When you learn to regulate your breathing you improve your overall health.

One of my favorite breathing techniques is called "box breathing." Close your eyes and picture a simple box. Visualize your finger touching the lower left-hand corner of the box and inhale for four seconds as you mentally move your finger across the bottom edge of the box until it reaches the lower right-hand corner. Hold your breath for four seconds as you draw your finger along the right side of the box. At the upper right-hand corner of the box, exhale slowly for four seconds while you move your finger across to the upper left-hand corner. As you head back to your original lower left-land starting point, hold your breath again for four seconds. Box breathing takes practice but can be extremely effective in calming nerves and regulating breath.

of a partner, we fear everything from the new normal our lives have become to the important questions we now need to answer alone. Kickboxing will help you face—and in some cases overcome—your fears as your spirit and confidence grow with each session.

There are fantastic kickboxing and boxing gyms popping up all over the world. Many gyms will give you a free trial, which will enable you to see if it's a good fit before you commit. Look for a gym with a community of like-minded individuals or with commonalities such as similar age, gender, or workout intensity levels. Also look for a knowledgeable coaching staff, which is critically important. You will want a coach who not only understands body mechanics but also fits your motivation style. Some people respond well to tough love, while others need gentle reassurance. Once you feel comfortable with a good coach you may find yourself brave enough to branch out into other forms of group exercise.

Zumba

Zumba is a form of group exercise that includes dance moves to upbeat music. I'm not much of a Zumba dancer myself, but I know countless people who love this type of training. You have active movement, increased endorphins, and great music to help your mood improve. Another benefit of a class like Zumba is you don't have to think about what to do next. The instructor plans the workout for you, and all you have to do is show up, participate, and hopefully have a little fun in the process. For those who love to dance and love to have fun, this is a great alternative to traditional exercises like running or weight lifting.

Zumba is also a great exercise for beginners because the workouts can be modified for your ability level, and the community you surround yourself with will laugh at the missteps and help you forget, at least for a short time, your worst pain. Zumba puts the fun back in fitness and offers a high caloric burn for most participants through its total-body approach. It can get you hooked on fitness maybe for the first time, and for many people that is a priceless side effect. One organized class of this form of exercise offers all the grief-coping tools I talk about most often. You get great community, upbeat and positive surroundings, full-body exercise that will improve balance and coordination, and fantastic cardiovascular stimulation all at the same time. For any person struggling with grief, Zumba can provide a needed escape from life's tough moments.

If you have social anxiety or aren't ready to be in a class setting just yet, Zumba videos are available online or for purchase. In fact, my online fitness program offers Zumba that can be done in the security of your own home.

Yoga

Yoga was a big part of my healing around year four of my grief journey. Before year four I felt as if I had to move and workout intensely to feel better. As I found my grief changing, I discovered I was growing and changing too. I felt like I needed more flexibility, so I participated in a hot yoga class to expand my fitness horizons. I loved the heat in the room, the flow of the moves, and the meditative state that yoga helped put me in. It was just what I needed at that particular time of my loss, and not just for the reasons I originally attended the class.

Yogic Healing

Culturally we are conditioned to ignore our mortality and deny our grief. Yoga helps us turn inward, process our pain, and in many cases release pent-up grief stored in our muscles through the use of stretches and poses. Yoga practices also teach the art of surrender, the art of cleanliness, and the ability to withdraw from the outer world. Yoga goes a long way toward improving not only our bodies but our overall lives.

Yoga helped me reflect, turn inward, and become still. The stillness was hard for me in the beginning—I didn't want to turn inward and hear my own thoughts—but as I grew, I knew I needed to listen more to my heart and embrace the things it was trying to tell me. If we are never still, then we can't hear what we need most at various times in our lives. Yoga can be a fantastic tool to help you start the process of self-reflection and personal growth.

Like nearly all forms of exercise, yoga is valuable for your mind, body, and spirit, and while many people may recognize just how restorative it is, it can be overlooked as one of the harder forms of exercise. Yoga is not easy. It is an excellent core workout that is challenging and often frustrating. You can gain tremendous strength and increase muscle mass, all while improving health. Yoga is extremely beneficial for improving posture, protecting your spine, and preventing cartilage and joint breakdown. Just like weight lifting, it can strengthen your bones because it is a load-bearing exercise, yet because you are using your own body weight, it is easier on your joints and tendons. Yoga also increases blood flow, which helps your circulation, especially in your hands and feet, as well as increases oxygen in your cells by boosting levels of hemoglobin and red blood cells, which carry oxygen to your tissues, helping the cells work better. I could go on and on about the benefits, from regulating your adrenal glands to lowering your blood pressure and increasing your immunity. Yoga is one of the very best forms of exercise you can do.

You may find that you need yoga earlier in your grief process for its restorative and meditative qualities. Since it is an age-old form of fitness and there are thousands of practices you can choose from, I would suggest you keep exploring until you find what practice works for you. Here are some of the more popular forms of yoga:

- **Hatha** is a great place to start. Typically, these classes focus on slow stretching and breathing. The goal of the class is to teach technique and help you learn to maintain poses.

- **Kundalini** is a very old form of yoga that just recently started being practiced in the West. The sequences are done rapidly and repetitively. This is a more intense form of yoga that is considered spiritual and mental.

- **Ashtanga** is a well-structured and advanced form of yoga made up of six different sequences. Each sequence has different characteristics and focuses on specific parts of the body. The seventy-five poses can take one and a half to two hours to complete and focus on detoxification, strength, flexibility, and stamina.

- **Hot yoga** is my personal favorite and is done in a room that is heated to between 95 and 100 degrees Fahrenheit with a humidity level of about 40 percent. Typically, this form of yoga is performed in a flowing style that links the poses smoothly. The heat helps promote flexibility and loosens your muscles. You will sweat and be extremely warm throughout the session.

- **Bikram** includes twenty-six postures performed in a ninety-minute sequence, and it often takes place in a hot room as well but not always.

- **Restorative** yoga can be particularly beneficial for anyone who is under stress since it focuses less on work and more on relaxation. Props such as pillows, bolsters, and even lavender-scented eye pillows are often used to help with relaxation. This form of yoga is a powerful way to recharge the brain, thanks to its restful nature.

Pilates

Pilates was created by Joseph Pilates as a rehabilitation program for World War I veterans. Its body-conditioning exercises are based on the fusion of body and mind with an end result of better posture, flexibility, and strength, and a positive transformation in the way the body looks, performs, and feels. Joseph Pilates believed in the overall power of the mind–body connection and developed precise movements that emphasize proper form and control over one's entire body.[1] There are six Pilates principles and philosophical foundations that place awareness on centering, concentration, control, precision, breathing, and flow.

Like most other forms of exercise, Pilates has strong health benefits, and like yoga it has a unique emphasis on the mind. Another benefit is that it encourages a strong back and core, the lack of which can often be the culprit behind many back, hip, and knee issues, common problem areas I see in clients. Pilates is a gentle workout that helps to preserve the longevity of the body. It also promotes body awareness through attention to posture both during your workout and through-out the day. As you raise your awareness of your body you will be able to change habits and relieve minor aches and pains, even prevent future body alignment issues.

Pilates can be an excellent choice if you enjoy yoga and a great way to build lean muscle if you can't take the intensity of weight lifting or running. Like every other form of exercise, timing and specific needs differ greatly from person to person. One person may find Pilates to be beneficial early on in the grieving process, while another may find the quiet and introspection difficult until much later on in the process. Only you will know what's best for you. Be open and willing to try all forms of exercise until you find what fits your needs at the various times in your life after loss.

Group Fitness and Community

I'm a huge proponent of group fitness and surrounding yourself with a solid community. Having a healthy fitness community was one of my saving graces while I was in the immediate throes of loss. Regardless of what type of exercise you decide to do, it is imperative that you surround yourself with positive and uplifting people. Make sure your community is one that will encourage you, help you grow, and push you forward. If your community understands the power of positivity, movement, and sweat, then you will go far.

I've seen thousands of grief support groups in my day, and many are beautiful, uplifting, and provide their members with opportunities to share with people better equipped to understand their pain. Some groups focus on bitterness and anger and do nothing more than to keep you stuck as you complain about what cannot be changed. Yes, you are allowed to have moments of bitterness and anger, but be careful you don't surround yourself with people who refuse to see hope and beauty. Your life will never be the same, but that does not mean it can't be wonderful. Surround yourself instead with people who empower your inner fight and fuel your fire for a new and better life.

Whatever you decide to do with your fitness routine, adding an uplifting community—such as the one you'll find at the Healthy Healing online portal—will help hold you accountable, give you like-minded friends, and keep you going on the harder days. When you feel like quitting or you stumble, your community will call you out lovingly, remind you how far you've come, and cheer you on. A positive community is worth its weight in gold, and when you find the

Sunshine, Vitamin D, and Earthing/Grounding

We are starting to learn more of what our ancestors knew instinctually, that we live on an electrical planet and we are bioelectrical beings. The concept of "earthing," or "grounding," might be an age-old concept, but it's just now gaining attention in the fields of psychology and neurology. Our bodies—the heart and the nervous system—function electrically and therefore need connection to our electric Earth. Emerging science reveals that contact with the ground allows your body to receive an energy infusion, compliments of Mother Nature. This infusion can have a powerful effect on your body by resorting and stabilizing the bioelectrical circuitry that rules your organs. Dr. Joseph Mercola, a leading advocate for personal health choices, writes, "The Earth carries an enormous negative charge. It's always electron-rich and can serve as a powerful and abundant supply of antioxidant and free-radical-busting electrons. Your body is finely tuned to 'work' with the Earth in the sense that there's a constant flow of energy between your body and the Earth.

"When you put your feet on the ground, you absorb large amounts of negative electrons through the soles of your feet. The effect is sufficient to maintain your body at the same negatively charged electrical potential as the Earth."[2]

It has been said that earthing helps boost self-healing mechanisms, reduce pain and inflammation, and even improve sleep and feelings of calmness. Couple your time outside with deep and cleansing breaths, and you may just find yourself refreshed and renewed for another day.

Another important part of being outside is that your skin gets some much-needed vitamin D. Skin and sun exposure has been cast in a negative light over the past thirty years, but according to dietary nutritionist Megan Ware, "adequate vitamin D intake is important for the regulation of calcium and phosphorus absorption, maintenance of healthy bones and teeth, and is suggested to supply a protective effect against multiple diseases and conditions such as cancer, type 1 diabetes, and multiple sclerosis."[3] Moderate sun exposure also helps your body produce serotonin, an important chemical that can help with depression. More and more, physicians and psychologists are recommending twenty minutes of uncovered daily sun exposure.[4] Sun exposure has been linked to cancer, but lack of sun exposure has also been linked to a rise in some forms of cancer. I realize this is still a controversial topic. I always recommend you check with your doctor and, more importantly, be an advocate for your body and your health. As a grief survivor, I find there is something especially healing about being out in nature and letting the sun warm my skin. Nature lends itself to hope and light, and during the darkest moments of our lives, hope and light are a tremendous lifeline.

right one you will know it, because those people will become part of your life forever.

Hiking / Nature

When I was a child, my father took me hiking all the time. Like any kid, I often complained about getting out into nature. As I aged, I started to enjoy the time with my dad and time alone in the quiet of a beautiful spot. As we hiked, my dad would tell me to be quiet and listen to nature because it had much to tell me. When we'd arrive at our destination he'd always stop and tell me, "Michelle, take a good look around. When you get off the beaten path you will see things most people in life will never have the chance to see. By getting lost in nature you sometimes are able to find yourself." Those words shaped me and helped define the kind of person I would become. There is no doubt about it: hiking and being outside in nature is uniquely good for the body and the soul.

It's obvious that hiking is healthy. You are most likely getting fresh air and some vitamin D, and you are moving your body, working your muscles, and clearing your brain. I've known for years about the restorative power of hiking, but science kindly backs this up. A recent study by the National Academy of Sciences concluded that "nature experience reduces rumination and subgenual prefrontal cortex activation." Essentially they found that more than 50 percent of people are now living in urban areas, and by the year 2050 it will be as high as 70 percent. With increasing urbanization, we are seeing an increase in our levels of mental illness. The National Academy of Sciences conducted a controlled experiment in which they investigated whether a nature experience would influence rumination (repetitive thought focused on negative aspects of the self), which is a known risk factor for mental illness. They had some study participants go on a ninety-minute walk through nature, and those people reported a lower level of rumination and showed reduced neural activity in the area of the brain linked to mental illness. This was compared to participants who walked through an urban environment and did not have the same positive result. The study concluded that a natural environment may be critical to our mental health.[5]

Just like with any other form of exercise, starting slow is key to safety and longevity when hiking. Purchase a quality pair of hiking shoes or boots that will suit the kind of hiking you will be doing. A good outdoor outfitter should be able to help you find the right fit and style for your personal needs.

A few words about hiking safety: Hiking can be one of the most rewarding forms of exercise, but it can also be very dangerous if you are not adequately prepared. Always research your hikes well, take enough food and water, never hike alone, and always make sure you tell others where you are going and when to expect you back. A little extra safety goes a long way when you head out into nature.

Other Forms of Fitness

I could add several additional chapters on other potential grief-coping forms of exercise—tennis, surfing, self-defense, team sports, and so much more—but hopefully the options in this chapter will help get you started on your fitness journey. Regardless of what you do, make sure you love it and make sure it becomes a daily part of your life. Remember, fitness is a means to more than just a better body; it's a means to a better life.

Whatever suggested exercises you decide to try, please just remember that as you move through your grief journey be flexible with your fitness choices. What serves you today and helps to give you strength and feed your inner fire may not last forever. One day you may need a flood of intense and powerful endorphins from running. Another day you may need the peace and tranquility of yoga or swimming, and a different day you may need to let go of the anger through weight lifting or kickboxing. Listen to your gut; it will reveal for you the way forward. Be willing to expand your horizons, try new things, and take chances. Be bold, brave, and ready to get off the beaten path. Just as your personality changes and grows through grief, so do your needs in regards to the exercises you choose. I will remind you of the important words I said at the top of this chapter: *Whatever you do, don't quit.* Just keep going and be committed to helping yourself through positive and life-affirming choices.

I'm proud of you for coming this far and being open to the idea of using fitness to help you move forward in your life. Regardless of who you are, we all face difficulties, and there is a power in taking back our lives, especially in a way that strengthens us for the journey ahead. It won't always be easy, but if you stay the course, find consistency, and move your body in a way that inspires you, you will feel the difference almost immediately.

CHAPTER 4

Nutrition

I often joke that someday I'm going to write a book about the crazier side of widowhood and call it *Don't Bring a Widow Lasagna*.

The concept of "comfort food" is familiar to all of us, not just those who grieve. We've all gone to our refrigerator and opened it up, looking for love, acceptance, happiness, and peace.

When you experience loss people often flock to your side, bringing you comfort food of all kinds. You are inundated with cookies, breads, pasta, and sugary pastries. The meal trains start out of the goodness of people's hearts and a wish to help. However, convenience food, while it looks good, often does little more than take up space. A grieving person may not be eating at all, and a meal train of food ends up in the trash or in the bodies of those individuals who are closest to the griever, including the children left behind. Most comfort foods do not nourish the body adequately and often lead to a vicious cycle of looking for happiness and love in all the wrong places. Food will not replace what was lost. Food will not fill the void, give you love, or move you forward. And yet food commands a powerful hold over us and dictates our moods, our sense of self-worth, and our feelings of strength and willpower. It has the ability to somehow comfort and destroy all at the same time, leaving us temporarily satisfied and happy but ultimately feeling weak or angry.

Food is connected with happiness, love, and fulfillment. Food makes us feel safe, and when we lose a big part of ourselves through death, we crave the security that was lost, the missing part of our soul. When we can't find it, oftentimes we look to food to fill the gap.

I wish it was that easy. I wish food could in some small way replace what we lost, but numbing yourself with food can only make your grief more profound, while you lose touch with your self-confidence and self-worth more and more.

It is important through this process that you remember food is neither good nor bad. You can and should enjoy your food, but you must stop giving food power over your heart and mind. Food does not have the ability to comfort, to fix, or to rectify. Food does have the capacity to satiate, to give strength, and to help regulate energy levels.

Food Is Not a Reward, Exercise Is Not a Punishment

Culturally speaking, we are taught from a very young age that food is a reward for doing a good job in life and a key part of our happiness. It's ingrained in us after sporting events when our parents take us for pizza, or when we pass a test or get good grades and are taken out for dinner. Summertime is filled with trips to the fair—funnel cakes, cotton candy, and ice cream—or vacations filled with vacation food, as much as we can eat. Our very happiness is tied to food from our youth, yet we wonder why we struggle with food addictions at a later age.

Food is not happiness. Food is simply nutrition for your body. Sim ilarly, I'd be remiss if I did not mention a key to your success as you travel forward:

Your fitness is a reward, not a punishment.

That one sentence made all the difference for me personally as I became One Fit Widow. Fitness is my time, and I love every moment of it. Fitness is where I go to release stress, work on me, and improve all aspects of my life. Culturally, we've been programmed to believe that when we eat "bad" foods (remember, food is not good or bad—it's just fuel) we have to exercise and punish ourselves with an hour or two of slow, steady cardio that we dread. We've also been told that exercise is just something we have to do to stay small and live longer. Let me explain that you just can't fix food choices with exercise. That's not the way it works. The size and, in many respects, the health of your body is determined by the food you eat. It's as simple as that. Stop trying to punish yourself for food choices with exercise, because exercise is an amazing gift to anyone able to participate. Exercise will help you feel more alive, process pain, and embrace the strength inside you. Exercise is not about making your body smaller but your life *bigger*. Think about that. Fitness is about making your life *bigger*. Wow, what a powerful concept. Fitness can literally change your entire life if you let it. Exercise is just that powerful, and you are forever going to remember it as your gift to yourself in this life. When you incorporate fitness, you have the chance to enjoy the depth and breadth of your world, and you have the opportunity to live truly.

The Grief Diet

Many grieving people put on a lot of extra weight after their initial loss. Comfort food is everywhere, and the endless bags of chips and cookies are a quick fix during the search for peace and a feeling of wholeness. You may subconsciously eat, looking for the piece of yourself that has been lost, without understanding that you are even more void of nutrients when you eat comfort foods. These foods hold no vitamins, no macro- or micronutrients, and leave the body begging for what it needs. For example, have you ever eaten an entire bag of potato chips and not felt full? Did you find yourself hungrier and craving a second bag? The potato chip companies are right: you really can't eat just one, because these foods have powerful chemicals and preservatives that leave your body craving more and your cells thirsty for any kind of real nutrients.

While many people numb their pain with food, others forget that their fragile bodies desperately need nutrients to survive the hardest days. In my first month after Mitch's death I lost a whopping fifty-plus pounds. They call it the "widow diet," and trust me it's no diet you want to try. I recall family bringing me a single egg each morning and begging me to eat it. I'd take a bite or two and push it away. Food had lost all its appeal; it offered nothing I thought I needed at the time. For months, pounds of food were dropped at my house, and I managed to feed my children yet hardly take in any calories myself. The weight fell off so quickly and so dramatically it had many people in my life concerned for my health. I didn't care, and weight loss was not my motivation. You see, my late husband loved food; he loved to cook and entertain family and friends, and so with his death I stopped enjoying the simple pleasures of a good meal. I didn't think about needing the vitamins and minerals from food; I just didn't have an appetite to eat. Like some people who overeat, I associated food with love, but instead of running to it, I ran as fast and far away from it as humanly possible.

Both situations—overeating and undereating—leave the griever completely malnourished. Both conditions are equally hard on a body that desperately needs good-quality and whole-food choices.

It is critical that you eat when you grieve, but it is equally essential that you eat well. I'd like you to take the remainder of this chapter to relearn everything you know about food. Consider how important it is, not only for your health but also for your mental and physical coping ability. When you eat less than optimal foods you get less than optimal results. When you eat large amounts of sugary foods you will likely feel sluggish and tired, and when you eat tons of bread and pastries you may feel sad and achy. I can't say how food affects you personally—we all process foods differently—but I can assure you that with better food choices you will be better able to face the hard days and nights ahead and may struggle just a little less with exhaustion and nighttime restlessness. Food can help in many ways, and my goal is to empower you to remember that with proper nutrition you can face the most difficult moments.

How should you fuel yourself during these tough times? Honestly, I have no different advice for you during your loss than I would for any client I'd share nutritional help with. Here are a few main points:

1. Make sure you eat enough food during this period because you need the calories for strength, especially since you will be incorporating in exercise as well.

2. Focus on eating *real food*. I'm sure you are thinking, *Isn't all food real food?* I'd argue that, no, not all food is real food. Skip the processed foods you see throughout every major grocery store. Focus on food that comes straight from the earth, the sea, or

the air. Think of it like this: if it can grow from or walk on the ground, swim in the sea, or fly in the air, and it is in its most natural state, then it's real food. For example, fresh vegetables, fruits, lean meats, nuts, and legumes are all real food. Just walk around the perimeter of any major grocery store and you will

The Eat-Sleep Solution

The grief cycle looks like this: limited sleep followed by a day full of extreme fatigue. You may fight the fatigue with sugary foods to give you energy and caffeine to help you keep your eyes open and do the things that used to come with relative ease. By nighttime you're sure you can't go on a minute longer and you lay your head down on your pillow, but your mind just won't let you rest. Thoughts go to loneliness, a to-do list that is miles long, and memories of what was and what could have been. You spend the night tossing and turning and wishing for just a few moments of rest. The next day you rise, jumping back on the hamster wheel and repeating the same habits that set you up for sleeping failure the night before. You're doing what you think you have to do to survive.

What if I told you that both food and exercise could help minimize that vicious cycle? What if I said that a healthy diet and regular exercise would make the highs less high and the lows less dark? I'm not saying they will fix the problem, but they can slow the hamster wheel and allow you a moment of bravery to jump off. Once you free yourself from the perpetual cycle, you may find that rest comes a little more quickly, and with rest you are better equipped to face a new day.

find where I want you to live. Load up on all the fruit and
vegetable colors you can find, and cook vegetables as minimally
as possible. (For a list of some whole foods to shop for, see the
"Healthy Healing Shopping List," page 245.)

3. Understand that some foods are known to have a positive
   effect on your emotional state and will therefore make those
   long days of grief just slightly more tolerable.[1] I will talk you
   through their nutrients in the next section. Focus on these
   foods as you do your grocery shopping and make meal choices,
   and you'll come to realize the simple but miraculous power of
   healthy healing with food.

Antioxidants

Stress is a major part of the grieving process. It would be nearly impossible to go through challenging life circumstances or the loss of
someone close without feeling the all-consuming stress that follows.
Eating foods that are high in antioxidants can lessen the damage of
free radicals often caused by stress. Antioxidants are deeply connected
to the prevention of cellular damage, the common pathway for cancer,
aging, and a variety of diseases.[2]

Examples of Foods High in Antioxidants

Foods with beta-carotene:[3] apricots, broccoli, butter,
cantaloupe, carrots, collards, egg yolks, liver, milk, peaches,
pumpkin, spinach, squash, sweet potatoes, tomatoes, yams

Foods with vitamin C: blueberries, broccoli, cabbage,
cantaloupe, citrus fruits and juices, grapefruit, kale, kiwifruit,
oranges, peppers, spinach, strawberries, tomatoes

Foods with vitamin E: apricots, fish oils, fortified cereals, nuts, seeds, vegetable oils, whole grains (especially wheat germ)

Load up on a variety of these foods to help your body better deal with the stress it's enduring. Just like fitness, this is not a "fix," but combining whole foods with all the other aspects of the Healthy Healing program will help you baby-step your way toward a stronger emotional state.

Carbohydrates

Carbohydrates are nothing more than the sugars, starches, and fibers found in such foods as grains, fruits, and vegetables. Carbs have a calming effect and can give your mood a boost through the chemical serotonin.[4] That being said, you must choose your carbs wisely. You will want to avoid foods that are high in processed sugars, like baked goods, highly processed breads, and cookies. The research is mixed, as is the case with almost all foods, but it does appear that the right carbs can have a positive outcome for at least some of the population. You will have to monitor and learn your own body's responses, which we'll talk about later in the book.

For years carbs have been the villain in the diet world. What we've learned over time is that all carbs are not created equal; the right carbs are not only healthy but essential for proper brain function and mental clarity, which can be vital when dealing with the effects of grief. To locate smart and healthy carb choices, focus your attention on nutrients and fiber content, which will slow your digestion, help with vitamin absorption, and keep your blood glucose levels more even. Typically, you can find these healthy and smart carbs in whole, plant-based foods, such as fruits and vegetables, and even in some minimally processed whole grains, such as oatmeal, brown rice, quinoa, and

Caution: Slow Down Ahead

A word of warning about eating a whole-food diet: incorporate any changes to your diet with moderation. Just like with fitness, if you make massive and sweeping changes, your new lifestyle may not stick, and you will find yourself falling back into old habits. Instead, take small daily steps and look to improve more each day, each week, and each month. I'm going to help you with that process in the coming chapters, but I'd much rather see you live a whole-foods lifestyle for 80 percent of your life than 100 percent perfection for just a few weeks. Perfection is not realistic, and the important thing is consistency rather than an unsustainable goal.

whole-wheat bread. You can also find smart carbs in beans, lentils, nuts, and seeds. (A more exhaustive list can be found on the Healthy Healing online portal.)

Examples of Quality Carbs

Beans (black, kidney, garbanzo, etc.)

Quinoa

Various vegetables (broccoli, brussels sprouts, cauliflower, eggplant, kale, onions, peas, romaine lettuce, spinach, squash, string beans)

Whole grains (barley, oats and oatmeal, whole-wheat pasta, etc.)

SIMPLE CARBS

What are simple carbs?

Simple carbs aren't all bad, and in some cases they are good for your health, such as when you're eating carbs full of fiber, like fruit. However, most simple carbs are found in highly processed foods, like the sugars found in syrups, candy, and soft drinks, which can wreak havoc on your energy levels and emotional state. Simple carbs often give you a quick boost followed by a downward spiral that leaves you low in energy and feeling sad. Watch your simple carb intake, and keep it as fresh and whole-food based as possible.

Examples of Natural Simple Carbs

Blackberries	Pears
Blueberries	Plums
Grapefruit	Strawberries
Grapes	Tomatoes
Kiwifruit	

Examples of Simple Carbs to Stay Away From

Cakes	Pies
Cereals	Sugar, both white and brown
Cookies	Syrups
Fruit juices	

Protein

The grieving body is often void of the nutrients it needs to remain strong and fit during difficult days. Protein—more specifically its building blocks, amino acids—is responsible for many essential health functions. Everything from your cells to your metabolism to your immune system relies on protein. So it seems intuitive to make sure your body gets enough protein.

Protein is not just for bodybuilders; protein is essential to maintaining and gaining new muscle mass, and eating protein at every meal helps the food last longer in your stomach and bloodstream, which prevents blood sugar crashes and keeps you "up" and alert for a few hours after eating. If you are not a vegetarian or a vegan, you will want to incorporate more fish in your diet, because certain fish—especially wild-caught fish—are high in mood-protecting omega-3 fatty acids. According to *Psychology Today,* "research has found that people who eat fish less than once a week have almost a third higher incidence of mild to moderate depression when compared to people who eat fish more frequently."[5] Protein, especially that which is coupled with omega-3 fatty acids, can be a powerful tool in the fight against the mood inconsistencies that come from grief.

Dairy is also a source of protein, especially some plain Greek yogurts and full-fat milks and cheeses, but I tread lightly with dairy and personally don't eat it at all. Try to avoid low-fat and nonfat products because they are chemically altered and filled with added sugars and preservatives. The healthy fats have been removed and replaced with dangerously high levels of processed additives, just to give the consumer the illusion of health. You would be much better off with the fats.

Legumes—another great source of protein—are also high in fiber, which keeps you feeling full longer and helps with digestive health.

Good Sources of Protein

Dairy products (in moderation)

Eggs

Fish

Lean red meat (bison)

Legumes (beans, edamame, lentils, peanuts, peas)

Nuts

Poultry

Seeds

Folate and Vitamin B12

Folate is one of the B vitamins (B9) and can be found especially in green vegetables, liver, and kidney. It is a key supplement for women of childbearing age, to prevent neural tube defects, but also it's been discovered that many people who are depressed have low folate levels. According to researchers Alec Coppen and Christina Bolander-Gouaille, who reviewed findings on major depression, "both low folate and low vitamin B12 status have been found in studies of depressive patients, and an association between depression and low levels of the two vitamins is found in studies of the general population."[6] Adding folate and vitamin B12 to your diet in times of stress or grief can pay dividends for your mental well-being. The good news is you don't have to run out and buy a folate supplement. So many great foods are loaded with folate. For B12, if you're a vegan or vegetarian, you may have to rely on a supplement, since so little B12 can be found in vegetarian foods, though fortified soy products and some cheeses contain small amounts of B12.

Good Sources of Folate

Asparagus	Lentils
Avocado	Liver
Beans	Mustard greens
Beets	Peas
Broccoli	Romaine lettuce
Cauliflower	Spinach
Citrus fruits	Sunflower seeds
Kale	

Good Sources of Vitamin B12

Beef	Fortified cereals
Eggs	Liver
Fish (mackerel, salmon, sardines)	Shellfish

Good Fats

We've been conditioned over the past thirty or so years to believe that fat is bad for our bodies, but in reality that is not the case. Fat is a necessary macronutrient and vital for good health. Fats, also known

Coach Tip

I *love* spinach, and over the years I've found it's super easy to incorporate it into my diet with some daily baby steps. Most days I consume 24 to 49 ounces of spinach alone. It all starts with my morning smoothie (see "Healthy Healing Recipes and Easy Meals," page 251); I consume 24 to 32 ounces in a quick and tasty drink. I typically add spinach to my egg scrambles or sweet potato hash, and it's a staple on my sandwiches, in my salads, and even alone, sautéed with ghee (clarified butter). I skip the iceberg lettuce and instead opt for nutrient-rich spinach in everything. Also, I have learned that it can be important to mix your greens for ultimate absorption within your body, so I don't hesitate to mix things up with kale, arugula (great flavor), or mixed greens. It's easier than you know. As you detox your taste buds in part two you will start to enjoy how it tastes and especially how it makes you feel!

as lipids, make up every cell in our bodies and aid in mitochondria health for strong and healthy brains. Dave Asprey talks about fat at great length in *Head Strong:* "A diet high in healthy fats helps to lower inflammation throughout your body and speed up energy production in your brain. The more healthy fats you eat, the more efficient your brain becomes at converting them to energy."[7] What we've discovered recently is that fats do many amazing things, including regulating our hormones, protecting our internal organs, and facilitating the absorption of vitamins.[8] Not to mention what they do for our hair and our skin. More importantly, and perhaps critical for anyone who is grieving, fats help us feel satiated and even boost our mood after eating.

Eating healthy fats, in moderation, does not make you fat and will help you feel better as well as raise your metabolic rate. Just remember to focus on unsaturated fats, such as olive oil, ghee, canola oil, fish, nuts, seeds, and avocado, for optimal health. Be especially vigilant to get your share of omega-3 fatty acids, which can be found in flaxseeds, salmon, chia seeds, and walnuts. Moderate your intake of saturated fats, found in fried foods, as well as many animal products such as beef, bacon, sausage, and full-fat dairy products like cheese and dairy desserts. Whenever possible it's also good to avoid trans fats, which are processed vegetable oils typically used in baked goods and commercially fried foods, such as french fries.

Stocking a Healthy Healing Kitchen

You will find a suggested shopping list later in the book (page 245) with recommended items to help you move toward a healthy and whole-foods diet, as well as healthy and easy-to-make recipes (page 251). The grocery list is not meant to be exhaustive. It would be nearly impossible to list all the foods you can eat during this program, and I want you to find comfort in that fact! Your choices are many, including foods you love. Also, no food is forbidden, because human psychology tells us that once we tell ourselves we can't have something, we start to want it even more. Instead, keep in mind that the foods on the shopping list will serve your body better.

Once you realize how valuable the nutrients you eat every day are for your grieving body, you will start to see the direct correlation between what you eat and how you feel. Food choices are about much more than simple taste or satisfaction. I want you to love your food and enjoy it, but food is also about the lasting effect it has on your body's daily output. What you put in will ultimately determine how you feel, your energy level, and even your susceptibility to common ailments like headaches. Let's explore this further.

Vitamins/Supplements

For the most part, I steer clear of recommending supplements and will instead ask that you speak with your doctor or naturopath about what your body may need. You could be taking something that is unnecessary while missing what you're deficient in. A naturopath can run a full blood panel and tell you exactly what you are deficient in, and some of those vitamins can make a big difference in how you feel.

Some Supplements to Ask About

BCAA (branched-chain amino acids)

Fish oil

Folate

L-Glutamine

Magnesium

Vitamin B complex

Vitamin C

Vitamin D

Tiredness

Being tired is a normal part of the grief process in many cases. The grief-stricken don't get enough rest, and sleep becomes difficult to come by. But what we often don't know or consider is that being tired can be a side effect of an iron deficiency. We can eat foods that are very good for us, such as beans, grains, and veggies, but the form of iron they contain is often weak and hard to absorb. "The National Academy of Sciences estimates that vegetarians absorb only 10 percent of the iron in their diet, while a diet that contains some lean meat, poultry, or seafood will deliver the average requirement of about 18 percent. Animal protein not only contains more iron, it's a special form called heme that your body absorbs better than it does the iron from plants such as spinach."[9] So if you are feeling especially tired you may want to eat a little more animal protein and a food high in vitamin C, such as citrus, melons, berries, dark leafy vegetables, or red or green pepper, which will help in iron absorption.

Irritability

Irritability can be a common theme with grief. Lack of nutrition and rest can leave you feeling sluggish and even angry. One thing that can help diminish irritability is giving up caffeine. Caffeine is a stimulant, and that can lead to irritable feelings, especially if you are already prone to depression, according to Larry Christensen and Ross Burrows of Texas A&M University.[10] Refined sucrose can also have this effect on people, and the two together can be detrimental to mood and energy levels (more on sugar later). If you think this is causing you problems, try giving up caffeine and sugar for about two weeks. If you feel better, add caffeine back in until symptoms develop. If you find yourself getting angry and irritable, consider cutting yourself off permanently. A good rule of thumb for me, because I love my coffee, is I don't drink coffee after two P.M. That way I still get my caffeine fix without allowing it to interfere with my sleep that evening. This is one of those times when you will have to trust your ability to read your own body, and it is worth paying attention to it to help you live better.

Alcohol can also lead to irritability because it is a known mood depressant. I suggest giving it up for an extended amount of time while you're grieving so it does not become a crutch or a way to numb the pain as you learn how to move forward.

Immunity Boosting Foods

The stress of grief and the inevitable exhaustion can often leave you with a compromised immune system, catching every virus and cold that comes your way. While food alone may not guarantee you don't catch a bug, it can certainly help boost your immunity and give you a fighting chance. Here are fifteen of your best food choices for a strong immune system:[11]

1. **Citrus fruits**—Grapefruits, lemons, limes, oranges, and tangerines are all high in vitamin C. Don't wait until after you've gotten sick to start taking in vitamin C; make sure you get enough every day to increase your body's production of white blood cells, which help you fight infections.

2. **Red bell peppers**—Citrus fruits usually get all the credit for vitamin C, but red bell peppers have twice the amount, ounce for ounce, and as an added bonus they have beta-carotene too, which is a powerful antioxidant and mood enhancer.

3. **Broccoli**—This is a superfood in every sense of the word. It is packed with all kinds of vitamins, such as A, C, and E, and has antioxidants too. You can't beat putting broccoli on your plate to help you build your best overall healthy body.

4. **Garlic**—This functional and tasty addition to any meal not only will help build your immune system through its heavy concentration of sulfur-containing compounds, like allicin, but also may aid in lowering your blood pressure and slowing the hardening of your arteries.[12]

5. **Ginger**—Just like vitamin C, ginger has been found to help prevent colds. In addition, ginger has been found to decrease chronic pain and may possess cholesterol-lowering properties.[13]

6. **Spinach**—This leafy green veggie is full of vitamin C and antioxidants like beta-carotene. Keep it raw for maximum benefits, but lightly cooking it may release vitamin A, which helps with a host of things, like vision, skin, bones, and of course the immune system.

7. **Yogurt**—The live cultures in yogurt help regulate your immune system and boost your body's natural defenses.[14] You can also get some extra vitamin D, which is very important to your overall health.

8. **Almonds**—Almonds are full of vitamin E, which is a key component in a healthy immune system. Because vitamin E is fat-soluble—which simply means it needs the presence of fat to be properly absorbed—nuts are the perfect carrier for both.

9. **Turmeric**—This spice has gained popularity lately for its many health benefits, including its use as an anti-inflammatory and in the treatment of osteoarthritis and rheumatoid arthritis.

Additionally, since you will be working out from this point forward, turmeric is said to help reduce exercise-induced muscle damage.

10. **Green tea**—Especially green, but also black, teas are packed with flavonoids, which are a type of antioxidant. Green tea has high levels of epigallocatechin gallate too, another strong antioxidant. Additionally, tea is a great source of amino acid L-theanine, which may help your body produce germ-fighting compounds in your T cells.

11. **Papaya**—This is another fruit I love because it is loaded with vitamin C. Just one papaya can give you 224 percent of your daily recommended requirement of vitamin C. Additionally, papaya is loaded with potassium and B vitamins, including folate.

12. **Kiwifruit**—One of my personal favorites, kiwifruit is loaded with nutrients, like folate and potassium, but it also gives you a good boost of vitamins K and C. Kiwifruit's other important contribution is that it may help guard against respiratory problems.

13. **Poultry**—Everyone wants a nice cup of chicken soup when they don't feel great, and some forms of lean poultry are in fact found to be especially high in vitamin B6, which is important in the production of red blood cells as well as dopamine and serotonin.

14. **Sunflower seeds**—There are countless nutrients in sunflower seeds, including phosphorous, magnesium, and vitamin B6. You will also get a good shot of vitamin E for added antioxidants and immune health.

15. **Shellfish**—Shellfish is loaded with zinc, and while zinc does not get all the attention other minerals do, it aids in a healthy immune system. Crabs, clams, lobsters, and mussels can help you get the zinc you need.

Sugar

There has been a lot written about sugar in the past few years. It is highly addictive, and thanks to the fat-free boom of the '80s and '90s and the boxed food revolution, we are consuming sugar, in all forms, like never before. I always tell my clients that sugar is the root of all evil, and that might be a slight exaggeration, but we are consuming pounds more sugar each year than our ancestors did just a few generations ago.

Sugar comes in many forms and often with many names, such as high-fructose corn syrup and sucrose. Sugar will never leave you satiated; you will always want more. It also makes you feel hungrier, and in time it deadens your taste buds so you are continually in a state of needing more sugar. I typically ask my fitness clients to steer clear of all forms of sugar for about three weeks while they detox their taste buds, and you should too. This can be a difficult request, as people almost across the board experience signs of withdrawal, ranging from headaches to fatigue to flu-like symptoms. I can assure you it is worth the time and effort. Also skip wine, processed breads, and other grains, and limit fruit during this time frame, or at least stick to fruit that is lower on the glycemic scale, such as berries. After the three weeks is over, you can start to add fruits back. My clients are always amazed at how good they feel and how much better food tastes!

Remember, not all sugars are created equal, and as you clean up your life, stick with sugar from fruit, whole grains, raw honey, and coconut sugar, which I enjoy in my coffee. Whatever you do, dump the fake sugars and diet sodas! You are far better off with real sugar over the chemical alternatives.

Don't Skip Meals

We've all been told that breakfast is the most important meal of the day. Once again, use your own judgment and learn the ins and outs of your body and mood regulation, but if you skip meals, you may find yourself irritable and even weepy while wondering what is wrong—until you realize you haven't eaten. When you do sit down and eat your mood stabilizes and irritability disappears. My daughter calls this effect "hangry." That's a mixture of hungry and angry, and as the mother of a tween girl, I can assure you it is a very real phenomenon. Eating regularly, especially first thing in the morning, will help normalize your blood sugar level, which in turn stabilizes your mood. Sometimes you may not find yourself hungry in the morning. I'd suggest making yourself a smoothie full of fruits and vegetables and the much-needed vitamins and minerals we discussed earlier in this chapter.

Intermittent fasting has become very popular recently, especially around the concept of brain growth. Learn your own body and study how different eating styles make you feel. I like what I'm reading about fasting, but I find it doesn't work for my body. When I skip meals I tend to gain weight, and I don't seem to benefit from the mind-clearing effects, so for me, eating small meals several times a day works much better. We will discuss in part two how to start the process of learning more about your body so any new fads that pop up don't have you confused and running down every rabbit hole. In the meantime, check out Healthy Healing Recipes and Easy Meals (page 251) as well as the online portal for my favorite recipes.

One thing I can tell you for certain: junk-food diets promote and worsen depression, and do nothing to help you create a positive and inspiring path forward in life. Diets that are high in processed foods, chemicals, dyes, sugars, and additives raise the risk of all kinds of health problems for not only your body but also your brain. People who eat these kinds of diets report higher levels of depression and anxiety in comparison to people who eat diets high in nutrients from vegetables, fruits, and lean protein. It's time we put the entire package back together. It's time we connect what we eat with how we feel. Eating right is not about how we look; it's about how we live. From this point forward, I don't want you to think of a healthy diet and lifestyle as putting limits on yourself but rather as making your life limitless.

CHAPTER 5

Getting Started

Starting is the hardest part of any journey. Starting is the thing that stops most people, but I don't want you to stop this time. Your health is too important, and so are you. In this book so far, I've told you my story and why it matters, and I've asked you to remember that your story matters too. I've told you about grief from my perspective, the judgment of others, and the importance of forward movement. I've also given you a little background on why I believe fitness and nutrition are a critical part of the grief-coping process and how I believe it can take you on a path toward healthy healing. Now I'd like to help you walk through the twelve-week program I designed.

Consider Healthy Healing a life-coaching program that will increase your knowledge, inspire a love of exercise, help you make healthy and whole-food meal choices, and remind you that your life from this point forward is in your hands and your control. I believe in free will and your power to positively shape your future. You cannot control what happened to you before this point in your life, but you can control from this moment forward how you react to it. This program will strengthen and empower you through the dark days ahead.

I'm not going to promise you that any of this will be easy, but I've seen the importance of healthy choices for thousands of grieving people, and I believe making these changes will help you too.

You will notice that the topics I cover and the homework I assign weekly should help you not only improve your view on fitness but also improve your life. These two things are not mutually exclusive. Your life and your fitness go hand in hand, so when you focus on one you are also focusing on the other. Fitness will make you stronger and more capable in everything you do, and it's well worth the effort it takes daily to maintain. When you focus on you, for even a short time each day, you will give to others more freely and live more completely.

Each week we will focus on a grief-related theme. I will offer guidance on how to cope with common issues, then we'll explore fitness methods, tips, and concepts as well as the basics of proper nutrition, which can be applied to not only to your life but also the lives of the people who are most important to you. These lessons will help you lead by example. Many of my personal growth homework assignments might seem simple and even like common sense, but I want you to remember that during a time of loss, it's best to start from a basic level. Simple steps, applied day after day, can lead you to some amazing places. I also want you to remember that common sense does not always translate into common action. Knowing what to do does not mean you will do it. Hopefully with the program's step-by-step approach you will find that translation into action easier. You don't have to leap. But even if you crawl, a year from now you will find yourself in a whole new place, amazed at all you have accomplished. Give this program twelve weeks and let it change your life for the better. I've seen it work for thousands of people and I know that it can work for you too.

Why 12 Weeks?

For a long time I resisted doing a multi-week program with my fitness clients because I believed it put too much emphasis on the short term and not enough on the long term. Fitness is a forever thing—the journey is the destination. You won't stay fit unless you continue to do the work, put in the effort, and make the choice to live differently for the rest of your life. One way I try to help people make the lifetime commitment to it is by reminding them that maintenance is an 80/20 proposition. If you can eat healthy, work out often, and live like a fit person 80 percent of the time, and 20 percent of the time you indulge yourself—while 100 percent of the time you try not to stress about the outcome—you will most likely be successful for life. Remember, this is a lifelong marathon, not a sprint.

When I eventually gave in and started a multi-week program with my clients, I learned that it helped them feel less overwhelmed. Laying "forever" out in front of most people stresses them, but a short-term, baby-step approach made it more likely they would start and perhaps stay the course. My hope is that once you start this program you will realize just how good your body is designed to feel, and you will want to keep going indefinitely. Once you dump the processed foods and add exercise to your life, and you get past the rough first few weeks, you will begin to feel amazing both inside and out, and that will give you the energy and the desire to keep going strong. It will be like somebody opened up the blinds on your life. Suddenly you will be full of energy, empowerment, and life, maybe for the first time *ever*. I consider this feeling a gift, and my hope is that you will open your gift and then share it with others. Together we can create a ripple effect worldwide for better and healthier forms of therapy.

Obstacles to Overcome

Perhaps you are already worried that you don't have the time, the energy, or the desire to make these changes and to do this work. You may be convincing yourself that time working on yourself is selfish, and everyone and everything else must come first. You may be thinking that because you love your kids, you shouldn't take a moment away from them, or because you are the sole breadwinner, you can't avoid working every free moment of the day.

I get it. I realize that it is hard for any grieving person to find free time during the day, and energy is usually very low, so this program may seem daunting. I also realize that guilt is a big part of grief. You feel guilty for being alive, for being occasionally happy, and you would feel even more guilty if you stepped away from work, your kids, your elderly parents, or any other pressing responsibilities to spend a second on improving yourself. Your feelings are real and genuine, but you can let go of the guilt because the people who love you most in this world would want you to be your best, to be happy, and to use Healthy Healing. They would never ask you to swallow your pain and ignore your needs. You shouldn't ask yourself to either.

Let me reframe this. Think about someone you love more than anything in the world—perhaps a child, a parent, or a very close friend. Do you want this person to take care of their health, be their best, and live a great life? Do you care about their longevity, their emotional health, and their physical well-being? Of course you do, and because you love them so much, you want them to do anything necessary to be their best. The people in your life feel the same way about you. It's time that you remember that and put yourself at the top of the list so you can be around for those people for a long time.

If you can promise me twenty to sixty minutes a day, I promise you will get that time back tenfold. You will become more productive, more efficient, and more capable than you were before. You will sleep better, eat better, and be better in all the important parts of your life. You will begin to optimize a life that has seemed impossible to juggle, and eventually you may even start to smile while doing it. The better you that you will become will have better relationships with everyone in your life. In essence, you will create time within your day by taking care of you.

Fat Loss, Not Weight Loss

Unlike many fitness and health programs, Healthy Healing will not focus on making you smaller or slimmer over the next twelve weeks. I always tell my fitness clients that I could not care less what they weigh; I only care how much extra fat they carry on their bodies. Weight does not make you unhealthy; too much fat does. If you are reading this book as strictly a grief-coping tool, the "fat loss" portion may not mean anything to you, but if you follow the program, you'll see that releasing the fat is accompanied by a more significant release, that of healing and renewal.

Since some people are also looking to improve their bodies as they heal, I'd be remiss if I did not touch on the fat loss aspect of the next twelve weeks. If you are choosing this program to lose weight while you become stronger and healthier, I'd like to remind you that the bathroom scale is irrelevant. Focus on making your life bigger rather than your body smaller.

As I've told you before, I believe every person and situation in life has something to teach us, or awaken in us, and I've seen it first-hand. I used to work in a gym where every Monday the clients had to "weigh in" before they left the gym. I'd watch strong, beautiful, capable women be reduced to puddles of tears in the bathroom because of the required weigh-in. Many of these women had just completed a strenuous workout that would leave anyone exhausted. They may have lifted a personal best, run faster than ever before, completed their first solo pull-up, or just walked in the door for the first time, but their accomplishments were diminished by a number that told them nothing of value. In many cases they'd leave dejected, questioning their hard work and buying into the concept that they are defined by something irrelevant. It made my heart hurt to see these people focusing on the wrong thing. Instead of being held up for all the things they were accomplishing, they were being defined by a number that had no relative bearing on their lives' true worth or meaning. Over the next twelve weeks, and for the rest of your life, I want you to remember that the bathroom scale does nothing more than provide a number

Nothin' but a Number

A number on a bathroom scale is nothing more than your relative relationship with gravity.

That's it.

The scale does not gauge your health, your happiness, or your beauty. The scale does not define your worth, tell you that you are loved, or share your spirit. The number is not tattooed on your forehead, and the number may make you feel happy and fruitful one day but defeated and sad the next. For the purpose of this program, kiss your bathroom scale goodbye for the next twelve weeks. Doing so will be key to your fitness freedom.

Fact or Fiction:
Muscle Weighs More Than Fat

When you start to eat a good whole-foods diet you inevitably drop weight. Couple that with solid exercise—especially an activity like weight lifting—and you will begin to add muscle quickly. A common misconception is that muscle weighs more than fat. Let me assure you that muscle does not weigh more than fat. A pound of muscle or a pound of fat is still just a single pound; however, muscle is much smaller, denser, and leaner than fat, and therefore takes up less space and creates long, lean lines. As you drop fat and add muscle, the scale may not budge at all, but your body changes dramatically as you become stronger and leaner in a matter of just a few weeks.

that is insignificant in the larger scheme of life. You know that now because of your loss. You realize it's not what really matters; it does not define your value.

Fitness and health are not about achieving some ideal of a perfect body but rather about making an excellent life. Think of this book as a chance to expand your horizons, to become better, wiser, more in touch, and more alive than ever before.

I'd also like to point out that fitness is only one part of how to cope with your grief. Fitness is a powerful tool, and I hope you use it to better yourself inside and out. I don't, however, want you to use it to escape or avoid your pain. Numbing can come in many forms, and fitness can lead to avoidance behavior as well. Any good thing overdone can have an adverse effect, so use fitness as a tool in your grief toolbox but seek other forms of therapy in addition to exercise. Myself, I love to incorporate music, nature, journaling, meditation, and of course proper counseling. Others find solace in drawing, animals, spirituality, and reading. How you move forward and heal is a personal choice, but having a good mix of positive therapies will help you continue to move toward hope and healing.

The list of helpful and healthy coping mechanisms is endless. Always listen to your inner voice, and remember that every new experience in life is a chance to grow and step into the next version of you. Every lesson, every loss, and every painful situation will eventually make you better if you allow the lessons to propel you forward. In my opinion, life is just one lesson after another. Some self-help gurus argue that it's not lessons but rather "remembering" or "awakening" to what we already know. Regardless of your viewpoint, being open to new circumstances will guarantee you a broader view of the world and your place in it. As you become wiser, you will begin to recognize these experiences, and you will start to use them to enhance your life. Death is the ultimate "learning" or "awakening" experience, so if you have been granted the opportunity to live beyond the loss of someone you never thought you could live without, you should be prepared for life to hand you something you never thought you could have. From a woman still standing nearly eight years after her loss (at the time of writing this book), I can assure you that life will be happy again, but you have to be willing to allow happiness to find you. You have to tell the universe you are ready to live again. You have to try.

All I'm asking for is twelve weeks. Are you willing to answer? If so, you're ready to take your first baby step.

What you'll be doing next may seem silly or strange, but it's a crucial component of your healthy healing journey. As I mentioned earlier, your weight is irrelevant to your success—it's the non-scale victories (NSVs) that count more—but a great way to see how your

Therapy and Counseling

Everyone in the world needs a good therapist. Regardless of your struggles, you need to talk them out with someone who is willing to listen and values your feelings. A good therapist will help you make sense of your feelings and embrace the evolution of your soul. A good therapist won't give you the answers but allow you to explore your own new emotional intelligence and find them for yourself. A good therapist can help with anxiety, PTSD, and the many other pains that accompany loss, all while normalizing the experience. Going to therapy does not mean you are weak; it is truly strong to face your pain, your fears, and your past so that you can move forward with your best future.

body is responding to your new, positive lifestyle is to grab a tape measure. You are going to start by taking and recording your measurements (see the following chart for where and how). I'd also like you to take photos of yourself from the front, the back, and both sides. Photos will be the best record of your changes, and even if it's hard to take them now, you will be so glad that you have them later. Trust me, I wish I had more photos of myself at 206 pounds because I'd love to look back at how far I've come. It's incredible to see subtle changes in your photos too, like a bigger smile and better posture. I always get told what a great smile I have in all my photos, and that compliment was never given to me before my fitness journey. Internal confidence, energy, and happiness shine out of you when you take control of your health and your life.

Measurements

To ensure accuracy, measure in exactly the same places and under the same conditions each time.

Week 1

Neck:

Chest:

Arms:

Waist:

Hips:

Quads:

Calves:

How to Properly Use Your Tape Measure

1. *Use the correct type of tape measure*—A soft cloth or flexible rubber tape measure like the kinds used in sewing is best. Avoid using a metal tape measure, as it will not be accurate.

2. *Stand with good posture*—Stand up straight and tall, and breathe normally. Some measurements may be taken more accurately when exhaling, some when inhaling—it will just depend on the measurement. This can be hard to accomplish yourself, so ask a friend to help.

3. *It is important that you measure correctly*—When you measure, make sure the tape is straight and in line

with each body part. For example, when taking your circumference measurements, make sure your tape is parallel to the floor, and your length measurements will need to be either parallel or perpendicular. This will be based on the line orientation of each body part being measured.

4. *Wear the right clothing*—It's hard to get good measurements when you're wearing baggy or extremely tight clothing, so aim to wear clothes that fit, or better yet, measure with nothing on.

5. *Write down your measurements and keep them safe*—Make sure that you write down the measurements as you take them so you don't forget them and need to take them again. Store them in a safe place you will remember so you can revisit your numbers later.

Body Measurement Locations

1. *Chest*—Measure the circumference around your chest at its widest point. For most men this will be at the armpits; for most women this will be at the nipple line.

2. *Upper arm*—Measure the circumference around the thickest part of your upper arm, which is usually at the center of the bicep.

3. *Waist*—Measure the circumference around your natural waist and your lower waist (two separate measurements). The natural waist is the smallest point of your waist (unlike where clothing waistlines are located these days) and is usually an inch or two above your belly button.

Your lower waist is the widest part of your waist, usually at the belly button or just below, where weight is generally gained first.

4. *Hips*—Measure the circumference around your hips at the widest point. This will be roughly just above the crotch line.

5. *Upper thigh*—Measure the circumference around your upper thigh at its widest point. This is usually half to three-quarters of the way up your thigh from the knee.

6. *Calf*—Measure the circumference around your calf at its widest point, usually three-quarters of the way up from the ankle.

Another great way to gauge your improvements will be through four specific exercises that will reveal your strength and cardiovascular improvements over the next twelve weeks. You will do a fitness assessment in Week 1 of the program, and I'd like you to pay attention to how much your fitness improves as you apply the program's methods and exercises.

Even if you don't want to dramatically change your body, you may be surprised by just how much exercise changes the density of your body. As your measurements change so will your energy level, your emotional strength, and your capacity to not only survive but thrive.

PART TWO

The Healthy Healing Program

Time Management

This first week's focus is going to be on setting you up for success over the next twelve weeks. You will be paying attention to what you eat because food will have a profound effect on how you feel, and when you feel good you can accomplish more. You will also write down your goals so you can keep your focus on why you started. And you will do a short fitness assessment so you can see how much stronger you become by the end of the program. Finally, you will dig deep to discover why you hope to use fitness as a grief-coping tool and why you've chosen a path toward healthy healing. But first, let's address the number-one concern most people face in the immediate aftermath of loss: time.

We all struggle with time constraints regardless of our various paths, and as a coach I've seen many people make time a roadblock between themselves and living their best lives. It can be a valid excuse, and I won't shame you for your lack of free disposable time. Looking back on when I became a mom for the first time, I remember asking myself what I did with all my time before I had kids. And after I became a widow, I remember wondering what I did with my time before I became a solo mom. Being a single parent and being a solo parent are two totally different realities. As a single parent you may have the support of the other spouse, who takes the kids half the time or maybe on weekends. You may have another partner to pick them up from school, run them to the doctor, or assist them with home-work. As a widowed parent, it may all suddenly be on you. It was for me, and it was overwhelming, to say the very least. I struggled with getting it all done. I struggled with time for myself and with the guilt I felt to be both mom and dad and do everything perfectly for my two innocent babies who had lost so much. Sometimes I struggled to remember that *I* had lost so much as well and needed time to myself so I could survive the solo aspect of my life after Mitch.

Carving out this time is not just therapeutic; it's essential. You can't properly process grief if you're in a constant state of doing for others. In order to grieve you need to make time for yourself every single day. Exercise is going to serve a multitude of purposes, including allowing you to grieve in your own way, process, and begin to move forward. It's also going to make you stronger, healthier, and better in all aspects of your life. There is no end to the benefits of a strong fitness routine.

I realize that time is not your friend when you live with loss, and I'm not going to pretend that this will be easy. Life is difficult and what you are facing is unfair. You are allowed to be overwhelmed and even angry. I get it because I've lived it. You are no doubt under extreme stress and you likely have no time for what's already on your plate, much less time to add fitness to your life. That being said, by fitting wellness into your life you will have more energy and process your loss in a much healthier way.

Time management is largely a personal choice. We make time for the things that are a priority. While death can alter your amount of free time, if you take an honest assessment of your day I believe you can find between twenty and sixty minutes throughout the entire day that you can use to improve your life. It's about reprioritizing and re-membering that a better you makes for a better life, because it causes a ripple of change that will benefit everyone you love. The best gift you can give to yourself and the people you love is the best version of you. If you are a parent, your wellness approach to grieving will teach your children more than words ever could about their own grief and the value of the days still to come. If you are a business owner or employee, your positive steps are sure to improve productivity and help relieve added financial stress. Plus, you will be showing friends and family that you prioritize your health, and when the day comes when they have to make a choice in grief—and we all eventually do—maybe they will follow your lead and take better care of themselves. Every aspect of life will improve in ways you can't always imagine when you begin to live a healthier life, and once you make that correlation you won't be able to *not* make time for your health.

Food Matters

I've told you how important food is, especially when it comes to your mood, but I've seen many people feel helpless when it comes to deciding what food is healthy. The entire concept of food has become too complicated, and I'm here to make it easy for you. You don't have to be overwhelmed, scared, or intimidated by food, and you don't have to give up the foods you love most. I'm simply asking you to choose foods that will support you and make you feel better, not worse.

You are what you eat, and your feelings and mood are a reflection of what you eat. That's why it's so important to me that you start recognizing what you put into your body and how it makes you feel afterward. Stop and consider for a moment just what food does for your body. Food helps cells grow, repair, and renew. Food gives energy to your body and clarity to your mind. Food makes up who and what you are, so if you are putting in the wrong fuel, you will not get good results. This is even more important for someone who is grieving and needing to even out the emotional highs and lows they are navigating. You may look in many directions for help with those difficult feelings, but the answer is right under your nose: the foods you eat. During Week 1, explore the recipes later in the book (page 251). You can follow the recipes precisely or use them as a jumping off place to improvise with any of the healthy ingredients listed in chapter 4.

Reading Labels

Because the concept of food is highly intimidating, start small and concentrate on not getting overwhelmed by the mass of information out there. During these first few weeks focus on one thing: doing your best to eat real, whole foods in their most natural state. As I previously mentioned, if it grows in the ground, walks on the earth, swims in the sea, or flies in the air, and it is in its most natural state, that's the sort of food you should eat. Aim to include fresh vegetables, fruit, lean protein, nuts, beans, and lots of water. Common sense, right? Not for everyone, and as I mentioned earlier, common sense does not always translate into action. We have become conditioned to eat food that comes quick and easy out of a box or a bag, but this food is void of nutrients your body desperately needs to help you survive life's biggest storm. Food is very powerful, and what you put into your body will largely determine your health through this process. You are already depleted emotionally and, in many cases, physically too. Your depletion can leave you vulnerable to illness and a more negative view of your reality. As you nourish the cells in your body over the next few weeks, you will start to feel "alive" in a new way. If you are conditioned to eat a highly processed diet, I think you will be incredibly surprised by how much better you will feel and how quickly. Truly, you have no idea just how good your body is designed to feel.

Cooking for One, or One Less

Cooking for just yourself, or cooking for fewer people than you did before your loss, can be emotionally daunting. I often hear the complaint that portions are hard to figure out and cooking at all is overwhelming. Remember to take the baby-step approach here as well, and make it as easy on yourself as possible. We are fortunate that nowadays stores and many restaurants prepare healthier options in smaller portions, and on the days when we can't bear to cook we can fall back on those resources. I'd suggest prepping some food ahead of time and always keeping your choices simple so mealtime does not become overwhelming. Some nights after Mitch passed I'd just grab a store-bought rotisserie chicken for my kids and eat some raw veggies myself. It was inexpensive, simple, and quick.

Your emphasis for Week 1 is to start looking at and considering the labels of the foods you eat most often. If you are eating *real* food in its most natural state as often as possible, then labels will not be the concern they were before, but given this program's baby-step approach, I'm assuming you will not be label free during Week 1. I don't want you to run out and buy a bunch of new food; I'd rather you to go to your refrigerator or pantry and start reading the labels on your boxed, canned, and bagged food. Look at the first several ingredients. Anything you don't recognize as real food in its natural state, plus any added chemicals, additives, and preservatives, will have a negative effect on your mood, your energy level, and your health. After the loss of someone you love, your chances of getting sick go up dramatically due to a weakened immune system, so let's do every-thing in our power to not only retain but improve your health.

Foods to Ditch

While you don't need to run out and completely revamp your pantry, there are a few ingredients you should toss out immediately:[1]

Sucralose, also known as Splenda, was never intended as a food product. It was originally believed to pass through your body without absorption, however the latest studies show this isn't the case. The pros are hard to find, so I'll just say that sucralose helps reduce refined sugar intake. The cons far outweigh that single pro. As you taste the artificial sweetener (which is the first con—it's not real food), your body prepares for sugar to enter the bloodstream. When it doesn't, the release of insulin in preparation for the sugar (assumed to follow) is left in limbo or released into your body, causing an excess of insulin. A third con is that it kills the good bacteria in your gut, and the loss of that good bacteria has been linked to disease and weight gain, includ-ing obesity. This is high on my "ditch" list.

High-fructose corn syrup directly caused the significant increase of sugar intake in the United States over the last thirty years. Cheaper than simple table sugar and easier to use, HFCS became a commonly used sweetener in our food manufacturing beginning in the 1970s. As its usage grew, so did the weight of the average American, increasing our obesity rates dramatically. Derived from corn, HFCS is the result-ing starch that sweetens our soda pop, candy, and other highly pro-cessed snack foods. Sweets, whether made from natural cane sugar or processed corn syrup, are highly addictive and have a serious impact on the health of the heart, teeth, thyroid, skin, body fat, and more. Sweets are also termed "nutrient poor" calories; alone they serve no nutritional purpose—a no-brainer when eliminating ineffective and unhealthy calories.

Sodium nitrate and sodium nitrite are chemical preservatives that slow the growth of microorganisms in prepared foods, extending the shelf life of the products. Regarded as carcinogenic due to their reaction to amino acids when introduced in the stomach, they are important additives to actively avoid, especially for children. Research has linked nitrates with childhood cancers. These preservatives are used in meat processing (bacon, hot dogs, lunch meat, jerky) and other processed foods. Meats are now available without either of these, except as naturally occurring. Watch your labels.

Hydrogenated vegetable oil utilizes a process that changes a liquid into a solid. This type of oil is yet another additive that preserves the shelf life of products (rather than the consumer!). Hydrogenated oil is the "trans fat" exposed many years ago by the heart health industry as a poison. You'll find a good number of products boasting "no trans fat" for this reason. This is a fundamental anti-health ingredient that is *not* GRAS (generally regarded as safe) by the FDA. That says it all. The FDA is notoriously slow to list an ingredient as "safe" or "not safe," so if they are hesitant on this one, you should be too.

Butylated hydroxytoluene (BHT) and butylated hydroxyanisole (BHA) are both used to stabilize fats—BHT to retain color and odor, and BHA to prevent the fats from going rancid. While regarded as safe (GRAS) by the FDA, they are on my list of additives to remove from your diet. BHT is still being studied for reactions in the body, and more and more studies with rats have shown BHA as a carcinogen. General Mills recently stopped all BHT usage in their cereals. Hats off to them, and it further supports that these, particularly BHA, are to be avoided.

Food dyes are artificial color agents used in a variety of foods, including—but in no way limited to—cereals, beverages, candy, desserts, cosmetics, and pet food. Sadly, a number of these products are marketed toward our children. Food dyes are linked to allergic responses, tumors, cancer, and hyperactivity and behavioral problems in children. In 2010 the European Union ended the legal use of these artificial colors and flavors. I hope the United States takes the same care in establishing what is safe to eat. In the meantime, be on the lookout for the three most widely used dyes in our food supply: Red 40, Yellow 5, and Yellow 6, which are all known carcinogens.

Your 12-Week Goals

Over the next twelve weeks I want you to focus on some achievable goals that you can chip away at weekly. Writing out specific goals is an important part of both your short-term and your long-term success and will help keep you on track. Think of these goals as a roadmap taking you where you want to go. For the purposes of this book, start with a few overarching goals in four key areas: fitness, nutrition, happiness, and personal growth (more on each of these later in this chapter). Nobody can tell you what your twelve-week fitness goal should be, but make sure you set your goal high enough that you have to work for it but not so high that it's unobtainable. All the goals create a vision and give you a measurable compass for your path forward. They force clarity, give life to action, keep you focused and motivated, and help you avoid procrastination. As you work your way through our twelve weeks, these goals will help you see all of the non-scale victories (NSVs) you have accomplished as you go. Seeing your positive results that aren't scale centric can be motivating and inspiring. NSVs can include lifting heavier weights, being able to walk or run farther, noticing more energy, or seeing your smile return in photos! Ultimately, setting goals allows you to measure your success and helps you feel accomplishment. In the following section you'll find prompts and

Defining a Clear Path

Make sure your goals are specific and detailed. The success behind written goals lies in you really thinking through the process and giving yourself as clear a roadmap as possible. Under each goal, it will help if you can write a short plan on how you will achieve the goal. For example, "I'd like to be able to run a mile without stopping by the end of the twelve weeks," and under that write the weekly action you will take to get you there. This can be a little time-consuming at first, but the success you feel later will make it all worthwhile.

space for writing your overarching goals for these next twelve weeks. (For a printable PDF goal sheet, visit the program's online portal at www.healthyhealingbook.com/healing.)

12-WEEK FITNESS GOAL

Your goals could be many things and are personal to you. Perhaps you'd like to run a 5K in honor of your lost loved one at the end of twelve weeks, or maybe you hope to hike a local mountain. Some clients have told me that at the end of the twelve-week program they were able simply to play with their kids at the park, and they found that to be a priceless gift.

Write your fitness goal here:

_____

_____

_____

12-WEEK NUTRITION GOAL

An example of a nutrition goal would be to cut out processed foods so you can be a good example for your family and friends, or perhaps you want to cut out soda or caffeine, which can be a daunting task! Your nutrition goal does not have to be complicated to be successful. Remember, so much of how you feel, how much energy you have, and how healthy you are comes from your nutrition.

Write your nutrition goal here:

_____

_____

_____

12-WEEK HAPPINESS GOAL

Happiness is so important, yet rarely do we put an emphasis on what makes us happy. We are so concerned with the needs of others that we forget our own, and that applies especially to people who are grieving. But if we make time for our happiness, we have more happiness to give. I also find that in our moments of happiness we often discover the inner parts of ourselves that still give our lives meaning.

Your happiness goal will help remind you that, despite your loss, your life is still valuable and you still matter. Some examples of happiness goals are going to see more live music or theater performances that bring you joy, taking up gardening, making time for get-togethers with friends, or simply laughing more.

Write your happiness goal here:

_____

_____

_____

12-WEEK PERSONAL GROWTH GOAL

I grew up with a father who did his PhD work in continuing education, so it's no coincidence that I strongly believe in lifelong growth. My favorite of the four goals deals with your personal growth journey. We do not make enough time for our fitness, nutrition, and happiness, and we certainly don't make enough time for our personal growth! Life is a series of lessons and growth opportunities, but often we are not open to the idea of growing, so we miss the experiences presented daily. Perhaps you want to go back to school and finish a degree, find your calling after your loss, start a blog to share your experience, or overcome the guilt that is holding you back from healing. There are a million ways to learn and grow in this life that don't require traditional schooling, and the more you open your eyes to the possibilities, the better you become in all facets of your life. Be open to various subject matters, teachers, and ideologies. You don't have to agree 100 percent with everything you read or listen to, but everyone you encounter does have something to teach you if you stop to recognize the lesson. Difficult people and situations can often teach you the most. Always remember to take what you need and leave the rest.

Write your personal growth goal here:

_____

_____

_____

WEEKLY GOALS

Now that you've set your overarching goals, I want you at the start of each week to set smaller, baby-step goals in each area to help you achieve each bigger goal by the end of the twelve weeks. For example, if your twelve-week fitness goal is to be more active, a baby-step goal might be to take 10,000 steps each day that week. If your twelve-week nutrition goal is to eat more vegetables, a baby-step goal could be to check out your local farmers' market and pick up exciting new produce for the week. If your twelve-week personal growth goal is to find some acceptance with the loss of your loved one, a baby-step goal might be to meditate three times that week, read a chapter from an enriching book, or listen to a podcast that offers insight. If your twelve-week personal happiness goal is to set aside one hour a day for yourself, a baby-step goal might be a daily ten-minute reading session or hot bath. I've learned that in both fitness and grief it is a good idea not to get too overwhelmed, and sometimes big goals can be scary. That's why it's important to break down your goals into weekly as well as daily actions. Before you know it, the twelve weeks will be over, and you will be so proud of how many life changes you've made.

Fitness Assessment

It's always a very good idea to do a "strength test" at the beginning of any fitness program. Remember, so much of your "fitness" will be more than just your physical strength. In the pages that follow, you are going to be working also on your mental strength and on helping yourself remember that life is still very much worth living. As you see your strength improve physically, take the time to notice how your strength in other facets improves too.

In regards to physical strength, you will initially test yourself in four different exercises: squat, mountain climber, push-up, and plank. (You can find video demonstrations of these moves, along with modifications for beginners or anyone with an injury, at www.healthy healingbook.com/healing.) For the first three exercises (squat, mountain climber, and push-up) you will count how many you can do within one minute; for the fourth exercise (plank) you will measure how long you can hold your plank. Set the stopwatch on your phone or keep track on a watch or a clock for sixty seconds while counting how many squats you can do within that time. Enter the total in the following chart. Next, do the same for the mountain climber exercise, with every time your right knee coming up toward your chest counting as one. Then count your push-ups, whether done on the floor, against a wall, or on an incline. Finally, hold a plank pose for as long as you can.

Don't forget to record your totals in the chart, because you will be referring to those counts at the end of the twelve weeks to see how far you've come. (For a printable PDF exercise sheet, visit the program's online portal at www.healthyhealingbook.com/healing.)

Week 1

Air Squat:

Mountain Climber:

Push-Up:

Plank:

Journaling

Writing is a wonderful form of grief therapy. Even if nobody ever sees your words, it is important that you get them out and onto paper. Don't judge what you write, and don't filter your thoughts. Allow your inner fears, pain, happiness, and dreams to make their way onto paper and into a higher place in your consciousness. Writing is cathartic and will help with everything from anger to sadness to loneliness to feelings that you don't feel safe sharing with others. In my early days of loss, and even still today, I was able to write my feelings with much more clarity than I could ever speak them aloud. Sometimes my honest and vulnerable words shocked even me, and the release I felt afterward was hard to explain. Once I felt brave enough to share my written words with the world, I found that my thoughts mirrored those of grieving people everywhere, which made me feel validated. Each individual journey is unique, but there are themes and threads common to all. Realizing I was not alone in my grief made me feel more normal and gave me a much-needed peace. We will talk later about a new morning routine that might include journaling, but for now, let's get you writing with your first homework assignment on your healthy healing journey.

Accountability Partners

Your goals are important, and so is some form of accountability. Within your twelve-week fitness goal I strongly encourage accountability partners to help you stay the course even on the days you don't want to. A good accountability partner will gently remind you of your goals, and help you get back up when you fall—and we all fall now and again. An accountability partner also will help you surround yourself with individuals who are going in the same direction. It's easy to be sidetracked by people who are stuck in one place, so now more than ever you need positive, forward-moving relationships.

Homework: Writing Your "Why"

Taking your health and fitness into your own hands is a conscious and deliberate choice, and it's often difficult to prioritize, especially for people who are grieving. Sometimes the work required seems formidable and unrealistic after life has taken a tragic turn. Like standing at the base of a fourteen-thousand-foot mountain, the journey often seems harder than we believe possible. What every good mountain climber knows is that you don't conquer the mountain in one giant step. Instead, you take a million small steps that lead you to a beautiful summit and a view few will ever experience. Once you reach the pinnacle of your health, you will realize that all the hard work, all the baby steps, all the sacrifice, was worth the effort, even if the journey was long and challenging.

I spent years thinking of fitness as a punishment for making poor food choices, or as something I had to do to look good or to fit into a certain size of clothing. Fitness for me was a superficial endeavor, and often that motivation was not enough to carry me through the hardest parts of the climb. Typically I'd go strong for a matter of days or weeks, only to slide down the mountain and find myself staring back up at the summit from the base. Just a few weeks before my late husband's plane crash I had slid back down the mountain of my fitness. The summit seemed farther away than ever, but I put on my gear once again and decided I was going to face the climb. My goals were the same as they had always been: losing weight, looking better in my clothing, and maybe having a little more energy to tackle my job, my kids, and my life. In other words, they were still pretty superficial.

After my husband's death, I realized for the first time in my thirty-six years of life that fitness was about much more than looking good.

I figured out that the key to health and fitness lay more in what I did with my life than in how I looked. I realized that fitness gave me new energy and new strength to face the impossible. It empowered me to face being a solo mother. It made me strong, inside and out. It saved my life. It was no longer about how I looked in a little black dress or a bathing suit. It was no longer about trying to burn off food that I probably should never have eaten. Fitness was not a punishment for how I was living my life. Fitness was a *reward* for being healthy enough to make the choice to live a big life. It was a reward for being alive and able to decide to make my life a priority.

All of these powerful realizations forever changed the way I chose to live my life and made me ask myself why. *Why do you want to be fit?* With this new enlightened perspective on health, I sat down and wrote myself a "why" letter. I took stock of where I was in my life. I noticed that my life revolved primarily around my two children. I wanted them to have their mother first and foremost. I couldn't control the future or what might happen to me, but I could manage my health and well-being to a large extent. If I made better choices with my health, then perhaps my odds of being with them longer would improve. Being a widowed mother of two babies, I realized that a goal like "being around" was now paramount.

I also wanted to lead by example for my children in all the most positive ways. Kids learn from what we do—not what we say we do. I wanted them to see me eating well, exercising, and choosing fitness as an everyday part of who I am. With my choices being healthy ones, perhaps my kids would make better choices with their lives too. Again, nothing is guaranteed, but I believe we most significantly affect the people we love when we model positive behavior.

Finally, I wanted to show my kids that we could all live life to the fullest. I had always wanted to be that mom who played with her children, who ran after them at the park. The mom who went down the waterslides, took them on hikes, and engaged in life in ways that helped them be bold, brave, and adventurous.

But my kids weren't my only reason in my original "why" letter. I also wanted to be fit for me, and I wanted to do it for my late husband. Death taught me so many things, but above all, it showed me how to choose life. It's not an easy lesson to learn, and there is no question that it's one of the most painful ways to learn, but if you pay attention, your life will never be the same—and often in beautiful ways—after going through loss. I realized that all the things Mitch and I had wanted to do, all the mountains we had wanted to climb, were still doable, but it was going to take my fitness to get me there. My hopes and dreams had changed and shifted with my loss, but I could still live an enjoyable life and fulfill many of the goals Mitch and I had laid out for our future.

My "why" became a catalyst for my fitness, and the "why" letter reminded me of all the reasons my health and fitness mattered. I found myself carrying on, higher up the mountain, even on the days when it was dark and stormy, even on the days I wanted to quit. My "why" was powerful enough to push me toward the summit. I still found myself tired and weary, but on those days I rested quietly, and instead of falling, I stood my ground until I felt strong enough to continue. What I also realized was that continuing up the mountain from the middle was easier than going back to the crowded base. There was no longer security at the bottom of the mountain; instead, I looked ahead to the thrill of a muddy and dirty trail on a path less traveled.

It's time to ask yourself why. Why do you want to incorporate a fit and healthy lifestyle into your journey? Why do you want to reach the summit of the mountain, and for whom does it matter? You may have convinced yourself that somehow it's selfish to take this journey, or you just can't spare the time away from your loved ones long enough to make it happen. You are probably overwhelmed with life—children, work, and keeping a roof over your head. Those items all take priority, but when you think about the people who love you most, all the people who rely on you and care that you are your best, you can't help but realize that those people want you to be happy. Those people would rather you take some time for yourself daily, even if it means losing a little time with them, because when you come back, you will be better, happier, and stronger than before you left. Quality over quantity. Happiness flows from happiness, so if you take the time daily to renew your joy, you will make those people around you happier because of the energy you exude. It may not be an easy concept to wrap your head around, but once you make the connection between your happiness and the happiness of the people you love most, you will forever understand that fitness is paramount to all aspects of your life.

So write your personal "why" letter because you just can't understand the value of this process unless you do it for yourself. *Yes,* this is important and, *yes,* you have the time. I want you to start by addressing the letter to yourself, and make sure you date the copy. Then list your reasons why, and get as deep as possible. If your mind drifts to smaller clothing sizes, a smaller number on the scale, or the way you look, stop yourself and start again. Go deeper. Remember, this process is *not* about diminishing the size of your body but rather enlarging the possibilities of your life. Your goal is not to shrink but to grow in strength, power, and hope. Your list should seem challenging but at the same time realistic. It should scare you enough to realize you are reaching for big things but inspire you enough to keep you going. This letter should be honest, heartfelt, and endearing. Go ahead. Write your letter now. I'll wait.

Now that you've written your twelve-week goals and your "why" letter, reread them. Do these things seem *big* enough to stretch your mind and body but still reasonable enough that you won't give up halfway to your personal summit? Does the list of goals inspire you to do and be more? Does it make you smile and encourage you to live truly? If you answered yes, then you are ready for the next step. If you answered no, then go back and edit ruthlessly! This is your life. Nobody can do this for you. You have to do it for yourself.

Once you are happy with your "why" letter, write your reasons why on a few sticky notes and place them around your house. Put them in places you will remember to look during this twelve-week process. After you have done this, then go ahead and put your "why" letter in a safe place where you won't necessarily see it until later on your journey. We will go back to your letter late in the program and give you a chance to reread your words, and edit them for a bigger and better future. As you improve physically, mentally, and even spiritually you will realize you are ready for bigger and better goals. With each reiteration of your "why" letter, you will start to understand that fitness is not a destination because you will never arrive at the top and stop. Fitness is a lifelong journey and forever a part of who you will become. Fitness will not only make your relationships with everyone in your life better but also improve your relationship with yourself, and that is the most important relationship you will ever have.

Guilt

I remember the first time I laughed after Mitch died. I felt so much guilt for feeling joy. How could I possibly find anything amusing or lighthearted enough to make me laugh? I remember the first time I felt proud of myself. I felt so much guilt for having a sense of fulfillment. I remember the first time I realized I could actually be happy again. I felt so much anger at myself for being happy. Happiness was in my past, or at least that was what I told myself. Being happy again was not allowed—I was a widow.

This week I want you to remember that guilt is a normal part of the grief journey, and there is power in accepting its presence in your life. You are not alone when you feel that guilt, and you are not alone when you get glimpses of happiness. Both emotions are normal, even healthy in some respect, because they show you the depth of your emotions and the complexity of loss. Don't let the guilt stop you from taking steps forward. Instead, accept the emotions as they come and face them with an attitude of personal growth and learning. You will learn from your guilt, and you will learn from your new happiness. Each emotion will help you build on the steps you are now taking to become who you will next be. As the weeks, months, and years go by,

Week 2 Baby Steps

FITNESS:

_____

_____

_____

NUTRITION:

_____

_____

_____

HAPPINESS:

_____

_____

_____

PERSONAL GROWTH:

_____

_____

_____

the guilt will slowly start to subside as you see the healing benefiting every aspect of your life.

Small steps are the key to your continual growth and success. Each week I want you to remember to write goals that are obtainable so you can keep on track toward the bigger picture. Please write this week's baby-step goals on the previous page.

Getting Past the Guilt

Guilt is very much a part of the grief process, and there is no way around it. It's an emotion that may seem senseless, but it's unavoidable for the grieving. The simple truth is, you will feel guilty. I wish I could take that fact away from you and tell you that guilt is optional, but it's not. And it's going to be important to your forward journey. Once you see that there is life beyond the guilt and it finally starts to subside, you will know that you are healing. In the meantime, let your guilt remind you that you can still feel, even if all you feel is the painful stuff.

You are also probably going to feel guilty for wanting to take care of yourself. It's going to seem selfish and self-absorbed, but I will continue to remind you that it is not. The person you lost does not have the opportunity to get fit, eat nutritiously, and be healthy—they are gone from your daily reality. Just that sentence may prompt additional guilt. That is not my intention, but it is just part of this process. They aren't here, but living your best life is a beautiful way to honor all that they were and all the love you still—and will forever—have for them. Living your best life is not something to feel guilty about; it's something to be proud of.

Guilt was a particularly hard emotion for me in the year after my loss. I was young and my life seemed far from over, but every time I did something "big" that reminded me I was still living, it hurt. This is the duality I spoke of earlier in the book. On the one-year anniversary of Mitch's plane crash, I took my kids to Aspen, Colorado, and showed them where we had lived earlier in our lives. It was one of his favorite places on Earth. He loved the mountains there and he loved the Roaring Fork River and Ajax Mountain. The morning of October 9, 2010, one year after his fatal crash, I hiked his favorite mountain to spread most of his ashes over a beautiful vista. In that moment I knew guilt was not serving my future life. No amount of guilt would bring him back, change what happened, or let me course correct. Guilt was simply keeping me chained to the past and regretting what was beyond my control. As I spread his ashes I started to let go of my guilt. My new life going forward was all I could control, and guilt did not have to be part of my new normal.

I want you to throw your guilt to the wind as you work through your twelve weeks. Forgive yourself for what came before, and take ownership of what comes next. Only you can.

Detox

"Detox" is a buzzword in the health and fitness industry. Countless people are selling detox shakes, pills, wraps, and specialty waters. We have this need to be healthy and fit *fast,* so we buy into the concept of a quick detox and even more rapid results.

The truth is, your body has everything it needs to detoxify and run efficiently. There is no reason to buy those expensive quick fixes because your liver and your kidneys do all the work on your behalf. Think of those products as only marketing tools, and remember that with the right nutrients and water, your body will do the job it needs to do.

For the purpose of this book, I'm going to refer to detoxing in a different manner. I'd like you to detox your food lifestyle, but I'd also

like you to work on detoxing other areas of your life: toxic relationships, negative thoughts, procrastination, preconceived cultural ideals
around grief and success. Life has handed you an unacceptable blow,
and you have the rare ability to see life from a new vantage point. If
ever there was a time to detox all aspects of who you are, it is now.

Let's start with detoxing your taste buds. It's not easy to do because much of our processed-food diet is full of sugar, sodium, and
preservatives. These additives alter the way food tastes, and over the
years you have probably become accustomed to highly sugary and
salty foods. People tell me all the time that they don't want to eat real
food because real food does not have as much flavor. I'm here to help
you see that the opposite is true. Fruits and veggies, nuts and legumes,
are bursting with flavor; you just have to reeducate and reawaken your
body's senses to notice it.

For the next week of your twelve-week program, eat as little processed food as possible (quick rule: if it has a label with ingredients
you don't recognize, toss it), limit your sugar intake (refined and
otherwise), and cut way back on salt. At first this is going to be very
challenging, and you may find that cravings are intense for about ten
days. You may even notice some adverse side effects, like irritability
and flu-like symptoms (headache, body aches, etc.). These symptoms
are pretty standard as your body readjusts to your new food lifestyle.
But soon you will start to experience a change in how food tastes.
Fruit may seem sweeter. Vegetables will be abundant with flavors
you never knew they had. You will also notice your cravings change
as your sleeping taste buds reawaken. A typical response is fewer
cravings for processed foods and a feeling of being satiated from the
nutrient-dense foods you are now consuming. Rather than craving
a bag of chips, you may find yourself craving a green drink or a bowl
of grapes. By the end of three weeks, you will likely start to feel
much better. The cravings will have completely dissipated, and you

will notice more energy and a real love and appreciation for whole foods.

I will never forget when I put myself on my whole-foods detox for the first time, and I sat down to eat a sweet potato. I suddenly realized why they called a sweet potato sweet! Until that point, my sweet potatoes had always been covered in butter or brown sugar; I had never actually tasted the potato. I was amazed at how delicious and sweet that potato was all on its own. The best part is that your body knows how to process a plain potato, and the food goes straight toward nurturing the body rather than the body trying to process synthetic junk. This nourishment is important because as you cope with your loss you will notice how taxed your body is from the stress, shock, and life-altering pain. Anything you can do to nourish your body will give you extra reserves to nourish your soul.

During this second week pay particular attention to the various foods you are eating and how you feel when you eat them. Do you feel satiated with healthier fats like avocados, nuts, or ghee? Do you notice any aches or pains when you eat dairy or grain carbs? Do you feel sluggish with protein or full of energy? Every single body is different, so it's important to learn how *your* body works. Think of this as an education in becoming the very best you, and your food is going to help you achieve that goal.

As you detox your taste buds, I'd also like you to work on detoxing your thoughts. Most people have heard the famous Joyce Meyer quote "You can't live a positive life with a negative mind." How much negativity do you allow via social media, television, or negative friends and acquaintances? If you allow negativity to come into your consciousness, then your life will continue to take on a more negative role. That's not to say you can't feel sorrow or stress, but the quicker you can return your thoughts to thankfulness and gratitude the more quickly you will find your anxiety decreasing and happiness seeping in. You will look at life differently as your new perspective changes the way you view the world around you. People's daily complaints and negativity will start to have an extremely adverse effect on you. Your tolerance for anyone who makes mountains out of molehills will diminish. Your tolerance for anyone who complains about the traffic, the line at the airport, or weekends of their husband watching football or golfing will bring up visceral reactions from someplace deep inside you that was awakened when your world was thrown on its axis. (And the terms "football widow" and "golfing widow" may make you feel anger you didn't know existed.) I'm not asking you to cut people out of your life, but carefully examine who and what gets your time and attention. You don't have to give an audience to people who focus on the smaller issues in life. You can choose to distance yourself from anyone who focuses on the negative, who is angry, petty, or not moving forward.

These negative types of people come in all forms and even sometimes in the form of grief group members. Find yourself a strong grief support system, but please pick your community very wisely and consciously. There are groups that allow you to be where you are, grieve in your own time, but also help you look toward the positive aspects of life. These will be invaluable to your journey. There are also groups that are based in anger, backward movement, and the concept of being a victim. Your loss is tragic and cruel and unfair, but it does not make you a victim to this life. Being a victim is a choice; instead, choose to surround yourself with people who want to rise up from the ashes. If you find yourself in a grief community that draws your energy downward, it's time to reevaluate and look for a group that will take your energy in a positive and uplifting direction. The people in this type of group will always allow you to feel your pain, but they will also celebrate your rebirth and forward momentum.

Warming Up Safely and Effectively

You've hopefully taken some baby steps to start exercising, or at least pondered which forms of exercise might be right for you. Great job! As you move through this program, one element of fitness will be key to your safety and success with your new lifestyle: warming up. Often people jump into their workouts cold, and they risk damaging their muscles, joints, and tendons. Regardless of what you do for fitness, make sure that you always appropriately and safely warm up your body before you begin. One of my favorite ways to have clients warm up is with dynamic moves. These moves should not be confused with stretching, which should be done at the conclusion of your workout, when your body is warm and loose. With a dynamic warm-up you increase blood flow and warm up your muscles, joints, and tendons as well as pay attention to your mind–body connection, clearing the neural pathways before getting into your workout.

You can jog in place, skip rope, or lift weights with low reps and very light weight. Rowing and walking on the treadmill are also great forms of warming up. As is key with everything in fitness, you need to listen to your body and never put more stress on your body than you can safely handle.

You may also utilize your warm-up to give you the mental strength to complete the actual workout. I know it's hard to get started, and some days you just feel like doing nothing more than lying in bed. By choosing a dynamic warm-up you are helping your brain and body prepare for and crave more movement. A little movement will make you feel better, and the warm-up might be all you need to keep going. During your warm-up listen to music that will inspire you to keep going, and remind yourself that this time is for you and part of your choice to heal in a healthy manner. Just ten minutes will most likely give you the energy to do another ten minutes, and so on.

There may be some days when the warm-up is all you can tolerate before you have to take a break, and that's okay. There is no judgment in this process. Promise yourself the warm-up and then see how you feel when you're done. I'm betting that the warm-up will make you feel better, and you will want to keep going, but I give you permission to start slow and work your way up. Healthy healing is not an overnight process but rather a lifelong commitment to yourself and your life after loss.

Homework: Gratitude Challenge

You've warmed up your body and detoxed your taste buds and the negative forces in your life. Now you'll focus on the biggest game changer out there: gratitude. It can be so hard to be grateful when you experience loss; you may feel anything but thankful. But gratitude for the small things and each of life's blessings can rejuvenate you when so many other things fail. Fascinating research is cropping up and giving validity to the idea of gratitude. There has been groundbreaking work in the past around consciousness and how we focus our energy, but science is now looking at these ideas from a practical standpoint and saying what motivational speaker Zig Ziglar told us: "Your attitude, not your aptitude, will determine your altitude."[1]

Gratitude takes practice and dedication, but with your new perspective you will start to see the law of attraction and the benefit of a new worldview. As you start to take daily note of what is good in your life, your consistent observation will have the power to make the good

Gratitude and Positivity for the Brain

There is strong science showing that gratitude and positivity change your brain. An emerging field of study that focuses on positive psychology highlights that science. Happiness and success expert Shawn Achor talks about gratitude and its benefits in *The Happiness Advantage.* In his bestselling book, as well countless classes and training programs, Achor defines seven important principles and patterns that can ultimately help indicate future success: "The Happiness Advantage—because positive brains have a biological advantage over brains that are neutral or negative." He also talks about "the Fulcrum and the Lever—How we experience the world, and our ability to succeed within it, constantly changes based on our mindset (our fulcrum) in a way that gives us the power (the lever) to be more fulfilled and successful." Out of the seven, my personal favorite is what Achor calls, "Falling Up—in the midst of defeat, stress, and crisis, our brains map different paths to help us cope. This principle is about finding the mental path that not only leads us up and out of failure or suffering, but teaches us to be happier and more successful because of it."[2] If you've ever wondered if your attitude can really make a difference to your future, you need to pick up this book and see the connection between the power of thought and the importance of gratitude.

more prevalent. At first it may seem like a forced exercise, as your focus is intent on what you've lost, but in time the gentle reminders of what remains will start to feel more genuine and sincere. Your positive energy will attract more goodness and manifest more happiness.

This week's homework is important to me personally, like so many of the homework assignments I will be giving throughout this book. Some assignments are more fitness related, and some have more to do with your life and how you face the difficult days. This one is vital because it is my belief that the more we focus on all we have to be grateful for, the more gratitude will appear. But first, let me tell you a personal story of the time I realized that gratitude was powerful and why I hope you pay close attention to this particular assignment.

As I mentioned, my late husband passed in early October of 2009, and just a few weeks later I was faced with my very first Thanksgiving without him. I went ahead and planned the holiday despite my horrendous grief because I felt it was important to carry on the tradition for our kids. I didn't feel very grateful, and I even had moments of feeling very resentful toward a holiday in which we are supposed to give thanks. But I felt it was my duty as a mother and a way to honor a man who loved to celebrate.

I woke up early, and before the day got too busy, I ran a 5K race with our kids and a few of my closest friends. I remember pushing our stroller over the finish line in just over thirty minutes—pretty good timing for a girl who had been out of shape just a few weeks prior. I think the grief pushed me forward, the exercise and sweat washing over me and helping me survive my first holiday without him.

After I crossed the finish line, it dawned on me that despite my recent lack of thankfulness I had so much to be thankful for. For every pain I was experiencing, countless people were experiencing much worse. Here I was, with two beautiful babies, a community that loved me, my health and fitness, and a roof over my head. I had had fifteen years with Mitch, and while I wanted more, I began to feel a sense of gratitude for what I *had* been given. I sat down that night and wrote out a list of everything in my life I was thankful for. It was long— longer than I thought it would be—and it reminded me that gratitude had made my heart feel better, if even for just a short while. Gratitude opened up for me an endless list of blessings, and with it, a small piece of me healed.

Writing down a list full of gratitude is very challenging when your heart has been shattered with loss. Like everything else in this book, I'm not here to pretend it will be easy, but I think it's a very important part of your forward path. My homework for you this week is all about gratitude and how you face each day. I'd like you to wake up every single day this week and find three things to be thankful for before you even get out of bed. Write them down, journal about them, focus on them, and watch your world change. Your gratitude for what is does not diminish the loss of what was. Your gratitude will not fix your pain or bring your person back, but your appreciation will make your life—here in the present moment—that much better.

It's hard to want life to be better after a loss. It's easier to sit in the pain and become a victim to your circumstances. But taking the "easy road" will find you twenty years later stuck, angry, bitter, and lost. You will look back and wonder what happened to your life. You will end up full of regrets and counting your excuses. I don't want that to happen to you. I want you to build your life in a healthy manner that takes you away from bitterness and toward thankfulness. Focusing on the good that remains will give you your life back.

Gratitude is just that powerful.

Nature and Quiet Time

Taking time to be quiet, to be alone, or to be still can be a difficult thing for anyone experiencing grief. Aloneness is something a griever is all too familiar with. But there is a difference between being alone and being lonely.

I will never forget taking my young daughter to Michigan Avenue in Chicago just six months after the loss of my husband. We stepped off the trolley onto the world famous street, a mother-and-daughter afternoon provided to me by my mother-in-law, who was babysitting my young son. On the busy street, filled with thousands of people rushing along with their busy lives, I felt a sinking and horrific aloneness. In fact, I can say with certainty I'd never felt more alone in my entire life, surrounded by thousands of souls. I remember feeling so small, so defeated, so sad. Everyone was busy, rushing about and carrying on with their lives, totally unaware of how shattered our lives had become. Being surrounded by others does not make you feel any less lonely, and in many cases it can make you feel even more lost and afraid. I experienced similar feelings at family get-togethers, where everyone's lives had returned to normal while I had been forced

Week 3 Baby Steps

FITNESS:

_____

_____

_____

NUTRITION:

_____

_____

_____

HAPPINESS:

_____

_____

_____

PERSONAL GROWTH:

_____

_____

_____

to rewrite my story in the middle. Even surrounded by people who loved me, who cared, and who wanted to see me return to "normal," I felt desperately alone. I also couldn't stand to be alone because my thoughts would drift and I'd inevitably be reminded of what was lost and how much I missed Mitch's daily presence in our lives. I couldn't tell you which was worse, being alone or being surrounded, because ultimately I was just deeply and painfully lonely.

Over the next few years I started to embrace my alone time. It wasn't easy, and like everything else associated with grief, it happened in phases. I began to realize that in the quiet I could figure out what I wanted for my future. Not the future I had planned with Mitch, but the future I would create without him.

This week I want you to focus on coping with feelings of loneliness and finding peace when you are alone. This new perspective will help you as you manage this week's priorities, including eating more, not less; bringing proper form to your Healthy Healing workouts; and finding time for happiness and personal growth.

Nature Therapy

Nature gives me a very different feeling from that of being surrounded by thousands of souls. When I take the time to travel into nature I feel alone, but I never feel lonely. Nature gives me time to reflect, quiet my mind, and hear my inner voice. It makes me feel small—not in an intimidating and overwhelming way, but in a grand and inspiring way. It reminds me of all the beauty this life still holds and all the joy I can still experience. Being in nature is a cathartic and healing experience that gives me the clarity I need to take bold steps in this life after loss. When I connect to the power of a raging river, the rhythmic pounding of the ocean surf, or the sounds of animals on a mountain trail, I'm reminded that I'm still here for a reason and it's up to me to discover what that reason is. When I summit a mountain peak I marvel at the grand wonder that lies all around me, and I force back tears at the power of my body and, more importantly, my will.

In one spontaneous moment, nature can remind us that our problems, while tremendous, will not be the definition of our stories, but rather a beautiful and instrumental step in our growth and develop-

Seasons

We are a product of nature.

In nature we have seasons. We have a strong winter, when animals and trees and other creatures go dormant and rest in the cold darkness. Winter is followed by a spring, when new life awakens and blooms, and all the creatures start to feel warmth from the longer days and the beauty of emerging life. Spring is followed by a beautiful summer, when all the animals and plants bask in the sunshine. Fall follows, when trees grow deep roots and animals store food for the upcoming winter.

To think you need to be 100 percent strong, warm, and resilient 365 days of the year is not realistic, nor does it follow the laws of nature. You are going to have hard days, cold and dark periods when you go dormant, and times when you need rest for the journey that lies ahead. You are going to have periods when you awaken, bask in the sunlight, and gain strength.

You are a product of nature and you are allowed your seasons. The key is to grasp each season, embrace what it gives to your being, and grow in the appropriate manner.

No person basks in the sunshine all the time, because the sun does not always shine.

ment. The mountains after all did not become grand, the oceans did not become beautiful, and the canyons did not become vast and wide without years of pressure, fire, and change. Nature is a metaphor for our lives after loss.

Beyond the obvious benefits of fresh air and inspiring, humbling views, being outside allows your body to soak up natural sunlight. Too much time indoors can hinder the body's ability to repair itself. Both darkness and sunlight influence hormone production in the brain and the all-important protein BDNF (discussed in chapter 2). Darkness triggers the production of melatonin, which aids in sleep and relaxation. Exposure to natural sunlight increases the production of serotonin, which is associated with boosting your mood, promoting calmness, and increasing focus. A lack of sunlight can cause dips in serotonin and potential increases in some forms of depression, like seasonal affective disorder (SAD). By taking time to be out in nature you are not only giving your mind clarity and your spirit inspiration; you are also breathing in cleaner, fresher air and providing a natural boost to your being.

Regardless of where you live, you can find beauty in nature. Every corner of the globe offers nature, and every time you take a quiet walk under the trees, through mountain shadows, or next to ocean waves, you are reminded of the force within. Start with a simple walk alone. Listen and you will be amazed by what you hear, deep from within your soul. Don't tell yourself that the area where you live isn't pretty enough to get out and enjoy; every part of our world can offer incredible beauty if you look hard enough.

Eating More, Not Less

What I'm about to tell you is key to the rewiring of your brain and the longevity of your health. It's going to go against everything you think you know about health and fitness, and it's going to seem completely counterintuitive to your success. I need you to hear me out and have faith in not only my education as a coach but also my personal experience as a formerly overweight person.

You need to eat *more,* not less.

Animals

My oldest child was just about to turn three when her father died. Like any caring parent, I rushed her to a therapist and figured we'd help her transition through her new emotions. That being said, kids grieve differently than adults, and traditional therapy was not needed at her young age. In lieu of seeing a counselor, we opted to have her start taking horseback riding lessons. She loves horses and couldn't wait to try. I started to notice a real difference in her on the days she spent time with the horses. Similar to how exercise empowered me, the horses seemed to empower her and give her a much-needed serenity and happiness. Animals have an incredible and kind way of helping us heal. They love us unconditionally, and they offer peace and joy. I've found, especially for my children, that animals can be one of the very best forms of therapy available, and they have the added benefit of teaching responsibility, promoting love for another being, and offering pure joy. Plus, it takes a lot of self-confidence to command respect and attention from such a large and powerful animal. With each lesson I could see my daughter's belief in herself grow, and her beautiful connection to the animal seemed to offer peace to her little soul.

Of course, when I say *more* I mean more of what your body needs and wants. I'm not referring to endless bags of chips or convenience-store donuts. I'm talking about foods that truly satiate you at a cellular level and give you the energy and substance to reach your goals. By eating more, you activate your metabolism, which allows your body to start releasing fat and using the fuel to build lean muscle and energy. In all actuality, you probably won't be eating more, but you will feel like you are because whole foods are full of fiber, vitamins, and micronutrients. It may seem like more to eat a big plate of vegetables, some lean protein, and perhaps some nuts, beans, or grains, but these foods are what your body craves, and they will ultimately reshape not just your body but your health and well-being too.

This week I challenge you to start figuring out how your body works most optimally. While working with my clients, I've noticed that many people do really well when they eat smaller meals throughout the day. My advice is to give it a try over the next several weeks and see how it works for you. Aim to eat small to moderate portion sizes every three hours, stopping after dinner and fasting until the next morning. Make sure as many meals as possible have some sort of vegetable and a small amount of protein, but don't be scared of your good fats and complex carbs. By eating this way, you will keep your blood sugar on an even level, your energy will stay more consistent, and you will be less tempted by the foods that don't serve your greater health and well-being. As you continue down the road toward healthy healing, you will need to keep your body fueled so you can tackle the harder days that are sure to follow. There are countless theories on the best way to fuel your body—everything from intermittent fasting to the Paleo and Zone diets. But it's most important right now that you just *eat,* and that is why I'm suggesting the every-three-hours rule. Later you can look at research about various food lifestyles, but remembering to eat and to eat *well* in the early days of loss is critical to your ability to process the moments when you aren't hungry or have just stopped caring. It's another baby step on your journey toward healing.

Proper Exercise Form

Good form during exercise is crucial for your safety and the longevity of your body. Don't think about short-term results; instead, focus on long-term gains. Reflect on the body you want to have when you are seventy-four and playing with your grandkids. Think about your mobility and the importance of your body's capacity as it ages. In our youth, we feel unstoppable, but overuse injuries and improper form can leave us permanently injured, especially in areas like our knees and our shoulders.

I love to use my dad as a perfect example of why this is so important. At the time I am writing this book, my dad is ninety-three years old and has been fit and active his entire life. When he was ninety-one, he fell and broke his hip and scared us all. Often that kind of injury at such an advanced stage can be deadly—everything from complications during surgery to infection to picking up something terrible while staying in the hospital. However, thanks to a lifetime of exercise, good nutrition, and proper form, my dad was out of the hospital and into rehab within the week. Rehab was set to last six weeks, but my dad was released in just three. He used a walker for a few weeks to regain strength and heal, and shortly after he was walking on his own again. Today my father is still walking without issue and even still drives. Your body is meant to last for life, and if you take care of it, you have an excellent shot of that happening. You don't want to train for just today; you want to make sure you train smart for life.

When exercising, always make sure you're using proper form so as not to injure or limit your body's ability to move. Also make sure you are using your full range of motion with each movement. Often our range of motion is limited due to an injury or just getting older. We need to keep good mobility with all our joints, tendons, and muscles as we get older. When we exercise we need to continue increasing our flexibility with good form. If you have bad form and add a load such as dumbbell, you will potentially injure yourself over time.

Some key points when lifting weights are to breath during the lift. Inhale just before you perform your lift and exhale as you move through the lift. Focus on keeping a neutral spine—not arched or rounded—from you head to your lower back. Pretend you have a broomstick attached to your back with your head, mid back, and lower back all touching the broomstick. Hold your core tight during your lifts; this will also help to stabilize your lower back to help prevent stress on it. Keeping your knees slightly bent will take pressure off your knee joints and allow circulation as you perform exercises. Remember, it is more important to have full range of motion and good mobility with your joints first, before you add any "load" during your exercises. It is key that you don't hurt yourself, but because you are using exercise as a grief-coping tool, it is even more important that you are able to keep training toward strength and optimal mental and emotional health. I want you to stay healthy so you can heal in a healthy manner.

Homework: Meditation in the Morning

It seems like either you're born a morning person or you're not. I was never a morning person before I started my fitness journey. I always woke up, especially after becoming a mother, feeling like I was already behind and always rushing.

This is not unique to grieving. I think most of us feel that way. We start our days behind the eight ball, running late and taking no time for ourselves. We feel stressed from the moment our feet hit the floor, and we are consumed with thoughts of what we should be doing for others. Regardless of whether it's work stress, kids stress, or the stress from grief, we start our day with all the wrong feelings and intentions, and it bleeds its way into our entire existence.

Turning your mornings around requires intentional changes in small forms. Just a few minor changes can end up shifting your entire day, taking you in a positive direction. My homework this week is intended to help you get your days off to a better start. This homework is inspired by Hal Elrod's book *The Miracle Morning,* which I highly recommend as additional reading for your personal growth. I typically did all of these things each day, but condensing them into the morning helped me make even more forward progress. This new routine won't always be easy, nothing ever is, but it can literally transform how you experience each day. It's as simple as setting your alarm thirty minutes earlier each day, and here's the key: do not hit the SNOOZE button even once. I realize this can be difficult if you aren't sleeping well, but if you dig deep and end the vicious cycle, it will become easier, especially when you start to see the obvious benefits.

Once you wake up, do the following:

1. **Stretch**—Lightly stretch in bed, and as you stand up continue to stretch for one to three minutes. Start the process of your body moving in a way that will benefit the rest of your day. Your stretch will start the blood flowing and allow you to focus on how you're feeling and your breathing.

2. **Drink water**—Drink an 8-ounce glass of room-temperature water. Add lemon if you can. Lemon has many health benefits,

such as jump-starting your metabolism and helping digestion, plus it tastes great.

3. **Read**—Grab a book and read for five to ten minutes, or listen to an audiobook if that's what you prefer. I personally love audiobooks, which allow me to process in a different way and don't tend to make me as sleepy. It's a very personal choice. Any kind of book is fine; just taking that intentional time for yourself can set your day off right. I like reflective and personal growth books in the morning; they help me achieve more throughout my day.

4. **Journal**—Grab a notebook and for five to ten minutes write whatever comes into your mind. Don't put any preconceived notions or judgments on your writing. You can write about what you dreamed about the night before, thoughts surrounding life after loss, special anecdotes about the person you lost, things that you look forward to during the day, or things you miss most about your special someone. The point is to put your feelings, thoughts, and intentions on paper. Journaling is a powerful way to get in touch with your inner emotions, and it helps you heal in a productive way. Writing can also be a great way to figure out your purpose beyond loss.

5. **Listen to music**—While you write, find some music that moves your soul, brings you peace, and motivates you to make your day a good one. I personally love classical and instrumental music during this time of the day.

6. **Meditate**—There are countless free apps that will help you start a meditation routine of just three to five minutes each morning (see the Healthy Healing online portal for a list).

Meditation is a great way to start your day and focus on what you want to accomplish or the mood you hope to set for yourself. It quiets the brain and helps you focus on your inner voice. It also helps with anxiety, fear, and anger. One way to think about meditation is to imagine the ocean on a violently stormy day with a boat in the middle of it, being tossed around by the harsh waves. Picture yourself diving down under the water several hundred feet to the calm water below. That is what mediation is like for your brain and body. Perhaps your mind races, never calming, and this is causing you anxiety—like you are being tossed about in a violent storm. If you can dive down with your meditation practice, you will find the calm that lies just below the surface of your immediate consciousness. If you can learn to start tapping into that quiet part of your brain daily, you will find more peace, more intention, and more growth for a confident future. Fair warning: meditation is like anything else, it takes time and patience to master, but it is worth the effort. Start slow (baby steps), and add a little more time each week. Before long you will wonder how you ever lived without the peace it brings to your life. Meditation is also very good for your brain. Emerging science is proving that meditation not only is relaxing and good for anxiety and stress but also helps brain growth and development. This is no longer considered some new-age fad; it's being practiced by some of the most successful people in business, like Arianna Huffington, because it really works.

7. **Validate and affirm**—Each morning, as an extension of the gratitude journal practice from Week 2, get a pen and notebook, think of three things you love about yourself, and

write them down. You are your greatest advocate, and you have to recognize your best qualities in order to find the confidence to continue to develop more. We all have things we are good at and we love about ourselves. It's time to focus on those positives so with time you can start to believe that you are unstoppable.

It may be difficult, but I want you to try not to talk or interact with anyone during the thirty minutes of this homework. Don't check email or social media or pick up your phone or computer. Take this time, while the world is still sleeping, and make it all about you. Take this time to regain power over your life. These thirty minutes will give you a chance to process, grieve, grow, and heal. It may be the only chance you get all day to simply be you and do what is best for your soul. Just like all the homework in this book, it will take practice and new dedication, but you are working on creating your best version of you, and that takes time.

WEEK 4

Comparison

As we go through the journey of life, we love to compare ourselves to others. One of the greatest causes of human suffering is comparison. We look at what others have achieved, their success, their assumed happiness, and we make ourselves miserable discounting our own history and life circumstances. The problem is we don't see the full story when we compare and make assumptions. We don't know the suffering other people have endured, the hard work they have put in, or the sacrifices that brought them to the place where they appear successful. Behind the scenes there is much more going on than we are aware of, and we spend our time comparing our résumé with one that has had all the painful growth moments edited out. This gets us in trouble and leads us to unhappiness. Social media has made it even more difficult, as we are faced daily with the best of people via media channels. People put up only what they want others to see, carefully ignoring the character-building moments that define how we live. As I mentioned earlier in the book, life is difficult for every human being—nobody escapes pain in this life—so keep your eyes on your own path and don't worry about what anyone else does to get through

Week 4 Baby Steps

FITNESS:

_____

_____

_____

NUTRITION:

_____

_____

_____

HAPPINESS:

_____

_____

_____

PERSONAL GROWTH:

_____

_____

_____

each day. You alone define your path, and a strong way to more inner peace is to focus on you.

This happens with our grief as well. We feel the need to compare timelines, pain, and forward progress. We ask who has it worse, who has more agony based on our individual kinds of loss and the length of our relationships.

But your pain is not on the same measurable scale as my pain. I threw the scale out a long time ago. When you measure or compare pain, you miss the opportunity just to love one another and support each other through life's hardest moments. I'm not here to measure your heartache, because my journey is different from your journey. I can't measure a road I've never walked, and you can't measure a path you've never taken.

I'm sorry you are in pain from loss.

I'm sorry your life has taken a twist that was not expected.

I'm done comparing misery.

Instead, I'm telling every person who reads this to go live on their own terms and by their own rules. Regardless of how you lost your future, your love, or your partner, do not let it stop you from making the most of the moments you have left.

This week you're going to focus on the only person you should compare yourself with: you. You will track your macronutrients to see how you're eating and what it's doing for your energy, and you'll log your food to become more aware of what you're eating from day to day. Finally, you'll read more about mobility and the importance of increasing your flexibility and range of motion as you progress in your fitness goals. Of course, this is not a competition, but by comparing your progress week by week you'll get the satisfaction that comes with steady improvement—and that's more fulfilling than any external metric.

Quitting Comparison

Not only do I want you to skip the grief comparisons; I also want you to skip the fitness ones. I see this all the time with my personal training clients. Somebody will have fantastic results and others within the group will start to feel defeated. It always breaks my heart when this happens, because as a fitness coach I can assure you that every person responds differently to a fitness protocol, and the only competition worth having is with the person you see in the mirror. Some people have further to go and therefore their results appear more dramatic more quickly. Some people have muscle memory that helps their bodies respond more quickly. Some people are more compliant and therefore have quicker results, and still others are just fortunate that their body cooperates in a faster manner. Those who stress about the success of others are discounting their own hard work, so I kindly remind them that each fitness journey is different and they must focus on the successes in their own lives. I also remind them that they need to look at their non-scale victories (NSVs), such as better posture, more overall strength, increased energy, greater happiness, and most importantly, focus on how far they have come, rather than how far they *think* they need to go.

I'm passionate about helping you squash the comparison tendencies, partly because I've unintentionally caused them myself. Some of the most heartbreaking emails I get are from people who say, "Michelle, what am I doing wrong? I'm not finding life after loss as quickly as you" or "I'm not doing this right. You are so much further along than me." When I read those emails and comments it hurts my heart because my journey is not meant to be a threshold of grief success (like there is such thing), but rather a simple story of one woman's personal journey. My way is not the right way; my way is nothing more than my way. So when you look at the grief journeys others are on, try not to compare them to yours. Try not to ask yourself what you are doing wrong or what they are doing right. Instead, look at each person you encounter as a teacher, both good and bad, and see what they have to "give" you on this journey of loss. Some will teach you love and resilience, and others will give you hope and a shared community that brings peace. During your journey you will also be faced with teachers who show you how you wish not to handle your pain. You will see negativity, bitterness, and hate, and those lessons can be just as vital as the positive ones. Remember, we all must come to the other side of pain in our own time, on our own path, and with our own lessons learned.

Macros

Let's switch back to the importance of food and discuss a breakdown of what is going into your body so you can start to discover how it makes you feel.

"Macros" refers to the three macronutrients protein, fat, and carbohydrates (as opposed to micronutrients, such as vitamins and minerals). There are very different views on what percentage of each macro you should consume daily, but I'm going to speak in terms of living your best life and achieving optimal health, not in terms of becoming a bodybuilder or running a marathon. Before I give you my recommended breakdown, let's talk about each macronutrient and why your body needs it.

Protein—Where do I start with the importance of protein? Let's be very clear: protein is a key component in your overall health and plays a vital role in nearly every cell of your body. Your body uses protein to build and repair tissues, build and maintain lean muscle mass, and make enzymes, hormones, and other important body chemicals. Protein also acts as a building block of bones, cartilage, skin, and even

Protein Sources

There are many sources of protein, including meat, fish, dairy, eggs, legumes, nut butters, nut milks, and seeds. You can also find moderate amounts of protein in vegetables like asparagus, broccoli, kale, potatoes, and spinach, and grains like kamut, quinoa, spelt, and teff.

I'd recommend trying to get your protein from lean sources. By using up all your fat percentage eating fattier meats like beef and pork, you will leave very little room for the good fats, like avocados, egg yolks, olive oil, and salmon. It's important to keep your fats varied, so keep your protein as lean as you can.

blood. It's not stored by the body, therefore you don't keep reserves in your system and must replenish your reserves throughout the day. *For your best health, 25 to 30 percent of your daily caloric intake should come from protein sources.*

Fat—Remember the '80s and '90s when we were told relentlessly that fat had to be cut from our diet? Remember the food industry selling us loads of processed "fat free" and "low fat" foods? Unfortunately, they added artificial sweeteners, dyes, and additives to replace the flavor lost when the fat was removed. The problem with this (besides the obvious chemical crap it left behind in our food supply) is that our bodies desperately need fat in some capacity. In her article "What Do Fats Do in the Body," Stephanie Dutchen explains, "It's common knowledge that too much cholesterol and other forms of fat can lead to disease, and that a healthy diet involves watching how much fatty food we eat. However, our bodies need a certain amount of fat to function—and we can't make it from scratch.

"Triglycerides, cholesterol, and other essential fatty acids—the scientific term for fats the body can't make on its own—store energy, insulate us, and protect our vital organs. They act as messengers, helping proteins do their jobs. They also start chemical reactions that help control growth, immune function, reproduction, and other aspects of basic metabolism. Fats help the body stockpile certain nutrients as well. The so-called 'fat soluble' vitamins—A, D, E and K—are stored in the liver and in fatty tissue."[1] At this point, I'm not sure many consumers understand just how critical fat can be to their overall health, especially its place in our vitamin absorption.

According to Harvard Health Publications, "Good fats come mainly from vegetable oils, nuts, seeds, avocados, and fish. They differ from saturated fats by having fewer hydrogen atoms bonded to their carbon chains. Healthy fats are liquid at room temperature, not solid. There are two broad categories of beneficial fats: monounsaturated and polyunsaturated fats. When you dip your bread in olive oil at an Italian restaurant, you're getting mostly monounsaturated fat. Good sources of monounsaturated fats are olive oil, peanut oil, canola oil, avocados, and most nuts, as well as high-oleic safflower and sunflower oils. Polyunsaturated fats are essential fats. That means they're required for normal body functions, but your body can't make them. So you must get them from food. Polyunsaturated fats are used to build cell membranes and the covering of nerves. They are needed for blood clotting, muscle movement, and inflammation."[2]

I have very little trouble getting enough good fats. They are everywhere and I love them. The list of foods containing them is long, and these foods are delicious. Change your fat source each day. If you love dairy, enjoy organic grass-fed milks and cheeses, but leave room for plant fats, like avocados, olives, nuts, and seeds. *I would recommend 20 to 25 percent of your daily caloric intake be healthy fats.*

Carbohydrates—This is yet another food group that has been demonized by the food industry. Suddenly everything is "gluten free" and we are avoiding carbs en masse. Many people cut carbs out drastically for a short amount of time, thinking they will be able to steer clear forever. They inevitably drop a lot of weight quickly, as is the case with most elimination diets, and then the day comes when they break the diet and eat an entire pizza or loaf of bread in one sitting. Their body goes haywire. Processing the once-eliminated food can become more difficult, and eventually more weight gain happens. To make matters worse, regret and self-loathing follow, the individual ends up beating him- or herself up over the missteps, and days or weeks of emotional eating follow. Unless you have a proven intolerance to gluten, I don't recommend you eliminate all carbohydrates, or any entire food group, from your body. Your body needs carbs for energy and clarity of mind. Carbs can be found in sugars, starches, and fibers. *My recommendation for carbohydrate intake is to aim for 50 to 55 percent of your daily caloric intake, striving for those carbs to come mostly from vegetables and fruit.*

These macronutrient percentage goals should be reached each day, not at each meal. It's best to have all food groups present in every meal, then boost a lack of any single macro with a snack focused on what's out of balance. One caution is with protein: at any given meal keep your protein intake just below a third of your daily goal to not overload your system's ability to process it effectively and safely.

Logging Your Food

This week I'd also like you to log what you eat, but not to count calories or restrict yourself. Instead, the purpose will be to observe your various macros so you can see what percentage you are putting into your body daily. You may opt to log your food in a free online calculator, like MyFitnessPal. Apps like this one make it quick, easy, and efficient for you to track your habits. They offer a chance for you to scan labels too, and their databases are packed with nearly every option available at grocery stores and many established restaurants.

Tracking these macros will be a real eye-opener and will help you make positive changes to your overall health as well as your mood. Once you see what you're putting in you can start to educate yourself on what your body has the most success with.

How Food Makes You Feel

One of the central aims of this book is to help you understand the correlation between what you put in your body and how you feel about your life. Because food holds so much power over emotions, it is essential to know how to use food as a tool during the grief process. Like everything else that has to do with health and fitness, I'm careful not to tell you that eating better will "fix" your grief; it won't. Healthy food is not a surefire solution, but it will help level off the highs and lows of your inevitable roller coaster of emotions. Your emotions will come, there is no way around that, and honestly I want you to feel those emotions.

You may be surprised at food's particular effects on your emotions. Strong sugar addictions can cause more physical and emotional problems than you may realize. Sugar may make you angry or sad, or give you physical side effects like headaches or cloudy thought processes. Food chemicals and dyes may cause joint pain or stomach issues. Perhaps malnourishment is causing you to gain weight as you continue to eat out, trying to satiate a body that is sick and deprived. You won't ever know until you take the time to observe and recognize how food personally affects you. Learn your intolerances, allergies, and aversions as well as how food interacts with your genes. You will have

Foods for Mood

There are some excellent food choices when considering your emotional health. Fatty fish is loaded with omega-3 fatty acids, which have been shown to reduce incidences of mental disorders, foods such as wild salmon. Whole grains give your brain glucose, which is a primary source of energy and helps regulate blood sugar spikes, which includes foods like oatmeal. Complex carbohydrates, such as chickpeas or quinoa, release glucose more slowly, providing steady fuel for the brain. Lean proteins like turkey and chicken are sometimes called "nature's Prozac" because they help keep serotonin levels balanced. Finally, leafy greens are important as well because they are high in folate and other B vitamins, and deficiencies in these areas are often linked with higher rates of depression and fatigue. The more you explore the foods you are eating, the more you will see the connection to what you eat and your overall mood.

foods that make you feel good and foods that make you feel horrible. As you walk this journey of life after loss, put the foods into your body that help you become the best version of you.

Increasing Your Mobility and Range of Motion

The emphasis this week for fitness will be on mobility and range of motion. As is the case with nearly everything discussed in this book for fitness, there is an application for grief as well. Mobility is defined as the ability to move or be moved freely and easily. Grief, in my opinion, requires mobility and the deliberate choice to move forward. There is no doubt that you've been asked to create a future you didn't plan. Creating a new normal, new plans, and a new future will require you to stretch beyond your current level of comfort. We sometimes go too far, pushing ourselves to get over grief too quickly or exercising so intensely that we injure ourselves. My recommendation is to increase your mobility slowly and over time, so you can eventually look back and be amazed at your new personal mobility.

Range of motion might not seem like a big deal when we are young, but as we age it becomes more and more important. In fact, I'd say it's one of the most important overall factors in our level of fitness. If you don't have good range of motion and mobility, you will find it harder to move, which in turn leads to balance issues, back and neck problems, and much more.

One place that most fitness professionals see poor range of motion is in the ankle. This can be attributed to several factors within our society, including more daily sitting, which ultimately ends up shortening our Achilles tendons, and wearing elevated shoes, which automatically shortens the Achilles as well. You will notice limited ankle range of motion when you do exercises like the squat. Often this is due to your shortened Achilles. Simple stretching exercises can be done daily to help. (You will find several examples of stretches at the Healthy Healing online portal.)

Another place where range of motion is evident is in our posture. We do so much work on our computers or texting on our phones, our shoulders end up rotating forward. You can work on pulling your shoulders back through exercises that are simple yet incredibly important as you age. Scapular wall slides can be done daily and are the best for opening up the shoulders and helping you stand taller. Simply stand with your back against a wall and your entire body, including your butt and upper back, touching it. Lift your arms into a 45-degree angle with your elbows and the backs of your hands touching the wall, then do a wall angel. Slide your hands up, while in constant contact with the wall, then slide them back down. Try this for ten repetitions.

Knee and hip mobility is also very important as we age. Your knees and hips have to carry you far in life. Take good care of them. For your knees, stand with your feet together and place a rolled up towel between your knees. Do circles with your knees both clockwise and counterclockwise, five circles in each direction. This will increase flexibility and lateral movement of your knee ligaments.

For your hips, get down on all fours and lift your right knee out to the side. Make a big circle with it, both clockwise and counterclockwise. Do this motion slowly for five to ten repetitions on each side.

Think of your body and your life moving forward as a practice in increased range of motion. Push yourself beyond a level of comfort while also safely expanding your ability to improve and grow. As you age—and we all do—you will care less about how much weight you can lift or how far you can run. Your mobility and range of motion will start to take center stage in your life, and you will be glad you focused on this key component of fitness. You don't have to spend hours each day; just a few well-timed moves can save you years of frustration.

Homework: Journaling How Food Makes You Feel

A few years ago I decided to start journaling about foods that changed my energy level, about my various aches and pains, and about reactions like headaches. I journaled for a few weeks and discovered that, for me personally, grains make my knees ache, processed sugars give me migraines, and heavy foods like pastas and breads make me sleepy. Through my personal evolution I discovered that I'd had a life-long dairy allergy, which explained many periods of extreme sickness that had gone undiagnosed. The dairy was causing extreme stomach issues, hives, and a myriad of other serious health issues, like acne and sinus infections. Once I cut out the dairy in my life, my health improved tenfold. During my self-discovery, I also learned that raw foods—like greens, veggies, fruits, and seeds—made me feel full of energy, happy, and ready to tackle the world. What an amazing realization to know that those healthy foods made me not only look better but also *feel* better.

My homework for you this week is to keep a food journal and watch the reaction your body has to the various foods you eat. Do you have any adverse reactions, such as headaches, a lack of energy, body aches, or afternoon energy lulls? Are there foods that make you feel better, less mentally foggy, more full of energy, or stronger? This may seem time-consuming, but don't use time as an excuse to not figure out what makes your body tick. Your body is your only place to live. Foods that you may have struggled to say no to in the past might become easier to walk away from when you make the connection to how crappy you feel after eating them. Take just five minutes after every meal, one to two hours after you've finished that meal, and take stock of your body. Start with your head and work your way down. Notice your energy level, your emotions, your stress level, and your happiness. I think you will find it is all interrelated, and this new information will help you as you walk your way through the grief journey.

WEEK 5

Rest

In the year after my late husband's plane crash, I hardly slept a wink. Typically, I'd be exhausted all day from a night of restless sleep, and I'd eat or drink whatever was necessary to stay awake and get through the day. As the night came I'd find myself restless and unable to turn off the screens in my mind. My thoughts would bounce between sadness for the loss of my husband, sadness for my lost future, regret, guilt, fear, and loneliness. The screens would multiply as I'd lay my head down to sleep, and I'd toss and turn until finally giving up and filling my time with some mindless activity till daylight. This pattern repeated for months, and the exhaustion added to my sadness, my brain fog, and my lack of motivation to live a good life after my loss. Most nights I slept less than four hours, awake until the physical exhaustion from my exercise routine finally helped me get some much-needed sleep.

I don't want this to be your experience, or at least I'd like to help you limit this all-too-familiar reality with some actionable steps toward better sleep. This week we will talk about the importance of rest during your recovery, both emotional and physical. We'll also explore another element to add in with all the hard work you're doing: rewards.

Week 5 Baby Steps

FITNESS:

_____

_____

_____

NUTRITION:

_____

_____

_____

HAPPINESS:

_____

_____

_____

PERSONAL GROWTH:

_____

_____

_____

You'll notice that this chapter is considerably shorter than the others. This is intentional. Use this week to rest, recover, and reward yourself for all the progress you've made. You'll go into next week with renewed energy for the road ahead.

Getting Enough Rest

You already know that sleep is critical to your health and your emotional and mental well-being, but rest days are also critical if you are training hard with your fitness. Fitness can be very addictive, and of all the addictions you can have, it is the healthiest option, but moderation is key. I'd love to see you be active every single day of the week, but that does not mean you have to train hard at every workout; in fact, I don't want you to. Sometimes taking an active rest day that includes a nice walk in nature is the best choice for a tired body. Other choices for active rest days include various forms of yoga (such as restorative yoga), a good swim, or a non-strenuous hike, all of which can help replenish your mind and body. Movement is still key on your rest day. I don't want you to stop altogether, but skip the gym or the boot camp class and let your muscles repair.

Sleep

Hopefully the exercise you've been doing has helped you hit the pillow harder at night. I can't stress enough how important this rest is to someone dealing with loss. The body repairs itself while you sleep; your muscles rebuild and your mind erases the data you no longer need. Lack of good sleep also can add to negative thoughts and self-defeating actions, can cause cravings for processed and sugary foods, can raise cortisol levels, and can make you insulin resistant, which leads to weight gain and a higher fat diet (and not the good kind of fat).[1] When you don't get enough good rest you stay on a hamster wheel, doing the same adverse thing day after day. But overtraining leads to more sleeplessness and injuries, so instead of burning yourself out with fitness until you quit, be smart: train two to four days a week and take several days of active rest.

Homework:
Reward Yourself

I'm not a very materialist person, but I have a personal weakness for new shoes. After I had been training for a while and really made my fitness a priority, I decided to reward myself with a nice new pair of Salomon hiking shoes and took a hike I'd been wanting to tackle. The shoes were fantastic and the hike was even better. That's when it dawned on me: All these years I'd been rewarding myself all wrong. Food was not a reward for being successful, but my experience of a great hike sure felt like a fantastic reward! While I love good food, and I hope you enjoy good food as well, it should never be used as a reward for the personal successful milestones in your life. Food is just food and it should not hold power over your emotions. An important way to start reconditioning how you look at the foods you eat is to stop using food as a reward in your life. This is easier said than done, and it will take practice on your part, which is why it will be your focus this week.

I'd like you to pick a goal that is related to fitness, nutrition, or moving forward with your life after loss and then think of a non-food-related reward to give yourself upon completion of that goal. For example, your goal might be to workout four times a week for a solid month, and once you do that you will buy yourself a new pair

The Benefit of Massage

Grabbing a massage is an excellent reward. We tend to place massage therapy under the category of "luxury" when really it has numerous health benefits—everything from relieving stress to increasing circulation to promoting better sleep to lowering blood pressure. Massage should be considered part of our total well-being practice. In addition to the health benefits, massage has a practical benefit for those who are grieving. Human interaction and touch are critically important to overall health. The first time I had a massage after the death of my husband I cried the most cathartic tears. It felt so good to be touched, and it provided me with a therapeutic cry that resulted in a lot of inner peace.

of workout shoes. Maybe your goal will be eating whole foods or journaling to help you find your way forward, and your reward is to complete a hike you've always wanted to do. Maybe your goal is to purge the closet full of the stuff of the person you lost, and your reward will be an acupuncture appointment or a massage to help you unwind after that difficult task. Your goal can be anything as long as it's a healthy goal that moves your life forward. The options are endless, but once you start to associate rewards with adventures, new opportunities, and moving your life in the direction you want to go, you become unstoppable. Your reward can be anything as long as it's healthy and non-food-related. Think outside the box with this homework, and have some fun. There are so many ways you can reward yourself that have nothing to do with going out for a nice meal or drinking wine with friends. Keep it fun, healthy, and inspiring so you want to do it again and again.

If you're up for it, post your rewards—and what you did to earn them—on social media with the hashtag #healthyhealing and at the program's online portal so our community can follow along and congratulate you on your success!

A New Normal

One of the hardest parts of loss is losing the future you had planned with the person who died. My dear friend Christina Rasmussen, who wrote the book *Second Firsts,* calls this phenomenon "invisible losses."[1] Invisible losses come *after* the initial loss, and these losses are often extremely painful to process. Everything from losing yourself and who you are without that other person in your life, to milestone anniversaries, birthdays, and graduations. You must re-create yourself—who you are without that person in your life—and create a new plan for your future. Our society tells us that the hardest part of grief is the actual death, but in many ways it's the invisible losses that never stop coming. In the early days it may seem like you are partly living in a parallel universe. You step back and forth between your old reality and your new reality, never fully existing in either world. Nothing can ease this process except time and forward movement. It's important to validate these feelings and understand that they are part of the process for nearly every grieving person. These feeling are not abnormal and you should not feel ashamed about them.

Now that you have five weeks of healthy healing under your belt, you will spend this Week 6 on setting yourself up for sustainable success, both in managing your grief and in achieving your fitness goals.

Week 6 Baby Steps

FITNESS:

_____

_____

_____

NUTRITION:

_____

_____

_____

HAPPINESS:

_____

_____

_____

PERSONAL GROWTH:

_____

_____

_____

This happens not through one single dramatic action but through everyday adjustments that make it easier to adapt to your new way of life.

Over time you will become accustomed to your new life after loss. Life can never go back to what it was before your loved one died, but you are learning to live a new normal and take it in stride. Your new normal includes parts of your old normal, but the backdrop has shifted and the photos are minus one important person. For the first few years you may see your life from a strange far-off vantage point. You may feel like an observer in your own world, watching from above. You may observe the life that once was, complete with the person you lost, while also observing the life that now is, complete with whatever came after—seeing it all, feeling it all, and yet somehow feeling out of place in both worlds.

Your new normal will ultimately include a knowledge you never had before. This knowledge will keep you balanced, centered, and ever aware that your time on this earth is short and relatively insignificant. This new reality enables you to live large, follow your dreams, and love in a way that can't be put into words. With great loss comes great perspective. You are able to feel more deeply, love more completely, and take each day in stride knowing that your problems are only as big as you allow them to become.

Eating Out

You may be at a point when you're ready to go out and do more social activities. In our culture, this often means a fun evening out at a restaurant. But I often hear from my clients that they don't feel like they can go out and enjoy dinner with their friends any longer because they are trying to live fit. I usually laugh and tell them that this is an excuse and that eating out does not have to stop them from

Halfway Point

The end of this Week 6 officially marks your halfway point on your twelve-week program. On the last day of this week take your measurements again. You can also jump on the scale, but in all honesty I wish you wouldn't. That number won't tell you how many brave new steps you've taken in your life after loss. That number won't tell you how incredible you are for taking back the power in your life. That number won't show you the true value of your actions so far and how difficult they have been. Instead, take your measurements and your photos and make sure you write down three to five non-scale victories you've had so far. Use the hashtag #healthyhealing on social media so I can encourage you on your wins.

	Week 1	Week 6
Air Squat:		
Mountain Climber:		
Push-Up:		
Plank:		

living a fit life. I fully admit that eating out can make eating healthy more difficult, but it all comes down to choice, preparation, and some basic common ordering knowledge. Eating out at your favorite local fast-food restaurant might not be the best choice, but even then you can make *better* choices than you perhaps made in the past. I want you to live an 80/20 lifestyle, and I want you to make this an everyday part of your life.

The first thing you can do before you go out is try to find a menu online. Being prepared will be key to staying with your program. Once you find the menu, look for the best options: meals like lean chicken (free of creamy sauces and breading), fish, veggies, and greens. Drink a fair amount of water while you're dining, and eat slowly—it takes about twenty minutes for your stomach to tell your brain you're getting nourishment. Avoid cream-based meals, fried meals, meals with heavy sauces, starches, and white-flour carbs. Look for meals with lots of color and foods that are full of fiber. One of my favorite go-to meals at any restaurant is a large salad filled with veggies and nuts and topped with my favorite grilled protein. You simply can't go wrong. You can ask the restaurant staff to skip the butters and the extra sodium, and most places will gladly oblige. Try not to feel bad or be embarrassed about asking for changes; you may run into an occasional disgruntled staff member or chef, but in seven years I've had nothing but kind and helpful responses to my modifications. The good news is that when you leave the restaurant, you will feel satiated, not overstuffed or sick. Your body can do amazing things when you load it up with the right kinds of foods.

Now, what about going out after loss? Do you find it hard to head out into the world or do you crave being out of the house and not being alone? Good news: it's just like everything else in the grief journey—it's a completely personal reaction and neither path is incorrect. I remember hating to be alone most days and I looked forward to any opportunity to get out with friends and just feel normal. It was a kind of escape, and it made me feel less lonely. On the flip side, I've known people who struggle to get out of bed, and the thought of going out repulses them. Try not to judge your personal journey and remember that in time life will take on a new normal. Whatever feels best for you is what you should be doing right now. Even baby steps forward can pay huge dividends for you down the road. Maybe start with a cup of coffee with a close, trusted friend and build from there.

Emergency Food Kits

To be successful on this health and wellness journey you have to be prepared. If you head into your week or out into the world unprepared you will set yourself up for failure every single time. You will find yourself hungry, far from home, and staring down the doors of a fast-food restaurant or convenience store or just looking in your pantry for the quick fix to your hunger issues. Remember, eating whole foods is important to not only your health but also your emotional well-being, so you need to be prepared with snack options to get you through until your next smart meal.

I keep food with me at all times. It is really very easy with a bit of prep. I carry small packages of nuts, like almonds, walnuts, and cashews, in my purse. If I know I'm going to be away from the house for a long time, I take precut veggies and pack them in a small cooler or a portable lunch box, like PlanetBox. I also take along pre-bagged portions of protein—chicken, turkey, eggs, or fish—or single servings of peanut butter, almond butter, or hummus.

Scheduling a "prep day" on the weekend when you can prepare your next week's food is another way to make your food choices easier. Yes, it is time-consuming to set aside an hour or two to cook your protein, cut veggies, and hard-boil some eggs, but if you do this prep work you will have much greater success at staying on track throughout the week. I typically cook several chicken breasts and turkey breasts, and several ounces of fish (I bake them with seasoning to keep them moist), and after they cool I bag them or store them in 4-ounce quantities (about the size of your fist), which can be used for either meals or snacks. I also cut and wash all the fresh veggies so they are ready to grab on the run. This prep day is also a great time to make some fresh hummus and salsa. Whatever you can do to make your week run more smoothly and help you stay on track will be time well spent. It all comes down to being dedicated enough to know you want to fill your body with good whole foods.

Homework:
Prep for Success

When I first started doing my Sunday prep of food I scratched my head and wondered why I had never done it before. I noticed a huge reduction in my stress level the next week, and it was so much easier for me to stay on track with my new fit lifestyle. The little extra bit of effort went a long way toward helping me feel less anxious and overwhelmed.

This week's homework is very simple, but I believe it's critically important to your overall success. Perhaps you're telling yourself that you don't need to devote any time to preparation this week and you plan to skip my suggestions. I'm not letting you off the hook that easily, because I know you will find that once you take that time for prep work, you will never go back. It takes less time than you think, it's convenient, and it will help your entire week run more smoothly. I have four kids, and without my prep day I'd spend every morning before school rushed, stressed, and inevitably caving in to my weaknesses with food. Instead, my kids can reach in the fridge and grab the precut veggies I washed on Sunday and the precooked chicken and fish. You can do this too and make your life easier.

This week after you load yourself up with great nourishing food at the grocery store, plan to take one to two hours to wash, cut, and dry your veggies and your fruits. My kids love colorful peppers, and it takes me so little time to make sure we have a week's portions in the fridge. If you eat lean protein, you can use that same time to bake or grill some chicken or fish. I suggest cutting them into 4-ounce servings and storing them in quick to-go containers for your ease as you walk out the door. I also prepare snack bags of nuts and hard-boil a few eggs. I can tell you that the weeks when I do this are less hectic and ultimately I feel much less stressed. (The weeks when I don't take the time end up being a hot mess!) If you want, take a photo of your food prep and use the hashtag #healthyhealing so I can congratulate you on your hard work and dedication. Yes, you can do this! Yes, you are worth it!

Community

We don't have enough community in our daily lives. We've created an existence that isolates us from other humans and has replaced that sort of contact with various forms of interactive media. I run a virtual training company so I know that online community can be very effective, but our company also strives to give people in-person opportunities because we understand the value of human contact. Loneliness can lend itself to isolation and sadness, and there is evidence to suggest it can even lead to premature death,[1] so it's imperative that you make time to add community to your life.

During the first few weeks after the death of my husband, I didn't feel like I could breathe unless I could talk to him. I could be in a room full of people who loved and cared for me yet feel like I was completely alone. If you are like I was, you are missing the person who made you feel whole, complete, and loved. You are learning to live again without their presence. While no community can replace the person who once occupied that empty chair, it can help you feel supported and loved during those dark days. One important part of a solid grief community is acceptance and normalization. Like I've mentioned, grief is something we culturally don't understand, accept, or even acknowledge, so it's helpful to have like-minded people who get it and validate you

Week 7 Baby Steps

FITNESS:

_____

_____

_____

NUTRITION:

_____

_____

_____

HAPPINESS:

_____

_____

_____

PERSONAL GROWTH:

_____

_____

_____

in your grief. There are common themes with nearly all people who grieve, and that vernacular will not have to be explained to anyone who has walked a similar journey. This week focus on finding your tribe, meeting new people, and bringing your fitness and supportive community together by signing up for a local race.

It Takes a Village

Motivational speaker Jim Rohn famously said, "You're the average of the five people you spend the most time with," and I believe those few words are genius. Your community matters. Your fitness community matters, your spiritual community matters, your business community matters, and I can assure you that your grief community *really* matters. Grief support groups used to be few and far between except in older populations, but thanks to social media, your options for local and international community have grown exponentially. When I started One Fit Widow in 2012, there were very few places for the grieving to go to find uplifting support. On Facebook alone, there are now countless grief support groups for all kinds of loss. However, not all groups are created equal. That's just one of the reasons why I created One Fit Widow: to empower and lend support to a group of people in need of a place full of hope. Just like you want to surround yourself with the very best in fitness and health, you will benefit from doing the same with a grief support network. Let's face it, grief sucks regardless of your network, but some groups take a more positive outlook. Some groups encourage you to live again, find your purpose, and discover a new you, and they don't discount your hard days but help you avoid being stuck there forever. A strong group will encourage your reflection, your personal growth, and your changes through loss. It won't judge your process, won't tell you that you are doing it wrong, and won't fault you for finding new happiness and new life.

Trust me when I say your community is everything, so choose wisely and love them hard.

Helping You Find the Right Support

Regardless of the type of community you are searching for—fitness, heath, or grief—your community should be uplifting, supportive, and never competitive. Life is hard enough without having a community that allows its members to talk behind each other's backs, adds additional drama to your life, or does not lend true support. You can usually tell these groups early on. Watch for negative comments or petty disagreements. If you see a competitive angle where not everyone is encouraged to achieve, then steer clear. In the grief world, there are countless organizations online (see Resources for some good options, page 265). Depending on who leads the group, you will quickly sense a tone. The tribe I've grown is all about fitness, health, and living your best life. We support one another, and we strive for everyone to live their best lives. People who feed off drama don't usually last long. Don't be afraid to try new groups by joining hiking clubs, volunteering to help others, or having conversations with people on social media. Yes, it is difficult to put yourself out there, but when you find the tribe you want to surround yourself with you will be so thankful that you were brave enough to feel temporarily uncomfortable. After all, the good stuff in life always happens outside our comfort zones!

Homework: Sign Up for a Local Race

A few months after my late husband's crash, I ran my first ever half marathon. By the time the race came along, I was in pretty good shape and excited to tackle this new challenge. I remember standing in the race corral beforehand and taking in the energy of the amazing people around me. There were older people, amputees, people with shaved heads either racing for someone with cancer or battling cancer themselves, and people you might not think were that fit based on their size but their hearts and faces screamed "Healthy warrior!" I was so inspired just to be in their midst. To know that each person was there to complete a healthy goal made me want mine even more. It was truly one of the most inspiring mornings of my life.

This week's homework may seem easy to some and daunting to others. I want you to sign up for a race in your local community. It can be a 5K, a mud run, a Spartan race, a hot chocolate run, or a turkey trot. The distance does not matter, nor does the name of the race. The important thing is that you commit to the race and you experience that life-changing moment when you cross the finish line. You can walk, run, jog, or sprint. This is not about winning the race that day but about winning the race in this life. There are few things more impactful for me than taking part in a race, and I want that same feeling of success for you. Don't you dare get intimidated! By committing to a race you will surround yourself with a strong community to train with ahead of time, and if you don't have an in-person community, make sure you join us online. And of course you will meet a new and inspiring community on race morning!

Once you sign up for the race, make sure you hashtag #healthy healing so I can cheer you on, and you bet I want to see your race day photos! You should also share the event with your Healthy Healing family at our online portal. I know I've said this before, but running is a true metaphor for life after loss. Even when it's hard, you keep going, putting one foot in front of the other, taking risks, being brave, and moving in a forward direction. Run—or walk—because you can and because your life after loss still matters.

Numbing the Pain

It's quiet. It's daunting. It's scary. The rush of emotions comes and goes like a wave that threatens to take you out to sea and toss you in the most violent of storms. You can be fine one moment, going about your new and disjointed life, and the next moment you can be fighting for air, wishing you had just a few minutes of reprieve from a pain so deep you can't believe your heart is still beating. Maybe it's a song, a smell, or a memory that takes you to that place, and your fight-or-flight reflex leaves you with pain too intense to bear.

All you want is relief. You crave it, you cry out for it, and you feel the anxiety, the pain, and the absolute void of loss.

By this week, you are in your second month of Healthy Healing and ready to confront the intense emotions that have been springing up throughout this process. You might also be struggling with that horrible affliction that creeps up after initial motivation and success: a plateau. This week you will face these emotions and challenges head-on, and channel your emotions into more intense workouts and strategies that will help you use the pain to grow.

Week 8 Baby Steps

FITNESS:

_____

_____

_____

NUTRITION:

_____

_____

_____

HAPPINESS:

_____

_____

_____

PERSONAL GROWTH:

_____

_____

_____

Working Through the Pain

Grief is perhaps the hardest of all human emotions. We tend to do nearly anything not to feel the intense pain, loneliness, and despair that come with it. It can become easy to fall back on quick fixes, distractions, and numbness to avoid feeling grief. When that wise man came to my doorstep on that fateful night I lost my husband and gave me his advice—to not numb my pain; to instead live it, experience it, and survive it—I knew I would never forget his words. Of all the things I hope you take away from this book, this advice is one of the most important.

I've spent many years helping people live again after the shadow of loss, and during that time I've seen them numb their pain through alcohol, painkillers, food, and other unhealthy outlets. It's another version of the hamster wheel that so many of us run on unknowingly day after day. We jump on the wheel at the very moment the pain is unbearable, and for that moment we feel better, we survive one more day, only to return to the hamster wheel the next day because the crutch is easier to hold on to than the unsteady path we must navigate without it. Numbness smooths over the hard edges and gives us temporary relief from the pain. It also becomes an unhealthy addiction, and years of life can be lost as a griever relies on anything that will help them not feel.

Pain must be experienced in order for you to move toward healing. If you numb the pain, you are simply postponing it for another day, and making it harder for yourself in the long run. The pain will come; you can't hide from it. Rather than numbing it, decide that you're going to face it head-on. Ride the waves and take each day for what it is. It might be hard to accept that this tragic thing that happened to you is going to make you better; you might think that finding something positive in this somehow discounts your pain or minimizes your loss. I can assure you neither is true. Grievers who wish to evolve into a better person go through an incredible awakening or "grief evolution." Your physical, emotional, and mental betterment does not minimize your loss or make it okay; it's simply a testament to what your loved one's life meant to you. By becoming a better you, you honor the best in them.

So I don't want you to numb the pain; I want you to evolve through it. I want you to grow and use exercise, nutrition, small baby steps, and personal growth to strengthen yourself to survive the intense moments. Recognize the new energy, the new life, and the new perspective a walk will give not only your body but your soul as well. When you sweat you will feel alive and open to the possibility of living again beyond devastating loss.

Increasing Your Workout Intensity

You are eight weeks into this new lifestyle, and I'm hopeful that you are starting to see the small flame inside your soul grow. Through fitness you are fanning that flame, empowering yourself, and finding tremendous strength for the difficult road ahead. You may even find yourself craving the solace that comes from a good sweat and looking to increase the intensity of your exercise. It is important that you listen to that need within your heart, but it is also important that you listen to your body. Any increase in your workout should be done gradually over time. Trainers call this process "gradual progressive overload," and it is an important part of training smart. Day after day, week after week, month after month, slowly increase your intensity. Don't come out of the gate sprinting, because you cannot maintain that speed forever, and at some point you will either injure yourself or simply burn out. I don't want either of those things for you, so it's important that you go slow, add a little bit each day, and continue on for the long haul. Your body needs to last you a lifetime. Your joints and your tendons need to be cared for. Train for the body and life you want twenty years from now. Train for longevity and train for inner peace.

That being said, you do need to continue to push your body and challenge yourself. Your muscles, joints, and tendons need to be stressed in order to strengthen and develop further. If you don't intensify your training over time your body will plateau and you will eventually stop seeing the results you are looking for. If you are exercising with weights or resistance, it is important (as discussed in Week 3) that you perfect your form before taking on any additional load, but once your form is mastered, stress your body with a little more weight during each workout. By "load," or "stress," I am simply referring to tension placed on the muscle fibers to essentially tear them so they can "rebuild" stronger. You can add load with your own body weight, bands, water, hand weights, machines, and simple equipment like medicine balls.

I always enjoy watching people intensify their workouts and find that fire endorphins provide. Sure, it helps you get in shape faster, but for the grieving person it serves a much greater purpose. The intensity will fill your body with clarity, purpose, and strength. The intensity often will change the way you look at life after loss too, because it alters how you face your pain. So by all means, add the intensity, add the load, and allow it to fill you with life. Just remember to add it slowly, listen to your body, and respect your needs physically, mentally, and spiritually.

HIIT Workouts

HIIT—high-intensity interval training—is all the rage in the fitness world right now because it's effective, quick, and dynamic. It's also controversial; many fitness experts are divided on its benefits and impact. Those who promote a high-intensity style of training do so for many reasons, one being that HIIT mixes it up and therefore limits boredom. Most HIIT sessions are twenty to thirty minutes or less, so they can fit into a busy schedule and still offer great results. Individuals who devote themselves to high-intensity workouts can see dramatic results in body composition—especially in fat loss—and can also see performance changes more quickly than traditional weight training and cardio programs may offer. I've personally seen incredible success with HIIT for not only myself but for countless clients.

The Science Behind HIIT: EPOC

EPOC—excessive postexercise oxygen consumption—is one of the most important parts of HIIT. EPOC is a term for what happens after resistance training or cardio training—or a combination of both—when your body continues to need oxygen at a higher rate than before your exercise began. This occurs because your body is trying to get back to homeostasis—its typical resting metabolic rate. Because your body wants to return to normal levels it will use additional energy as it tries to replace the oxygen deficiency caused by exercising.[1] What that means for your body, in a nutshell, is that you will continue to utilize energy—in the form of calories burned—long after your workout is completed. When you train using a high-intensity style of exercise you drive the effect of EPOC higher than what occurs after traditional forms of exercise, creating a larger oxygen deficiency from the intensified effort.

Here's the very best part: the more intense your workout (not duration), the greater the EPOC and the greater the calories burned. How long after your workout does this last? Well, experts agree that the "afterburn" can last as long as twenty-four hours post-workout—

Intensifying Your Workouts

For sample HIIT workouts you can try at home, go to the Healthy Healing online portal. Feel free to do these workouts several times throughout each day, as a break from work or as a chance to just move! Remember, the added movement will clear out the brain fog and give you energy to complete your tasks. But you're not limited to only these moves to up the intensity—use your imagination! You can increase intensity by walking or running faster for twenty to forty-five seconds and then slowing it down for an active recovery over ten to twenty seconds and repeating that cycle. This can be done with nearly any movement, from swimming to rowing to elliptical and more. You are only limited by your inner fire for change.

twenty-four hours! Not all workouts will yield that kind of EPOC, but it's exciting to know the potential of return on a great effort.[2]

Calorie-burning (the least of our worries in this book) isn't the only benefit of an HIIT workout. Your brain and heart benefit as well. According to Dave Asprey, author of *Head Strong,* your cardiac fitness improves as well when you add HIIT to your exercise protocol. This is measured by the improved ejection fraction: "the amount of blood your heart can pump in a single beat." He writes that, "unfortunately, most medium-intensity cardio workouts actually decrease your ejection fraction. The best way to increase it is through running intervals, such as 400-meter sprints. The normal protocol is to run as fast as you can for 400 meters, walk for a minute as you recover, and then repeat the process until you can't run anymore."[3]

HIIT is also one of the best ways to help your body release endorphins, which will have a very positive effect on your mood, making all the effort worth it!

Don't Just Sweat—Build!

Many people assume that HIIT is all about doing cardio, but that's just not so. You can do HIIT with just about any combination of exercises, including strength training. The old-school rules said that if you wanted fat loss you had to center your training on long, slow cardiorespiratory activities, like cycling, using the StairMaster, or jogging. Now, that's not to say those exercises do not have value—because they do—but that value pales in comparison to resistance training.

Why? The answer is simple. Resistance training builds lean muscle, and lean muscle helps you gain strength, drop fat, and lose inches. It's also metabolically active, which means it takes a ton of energy to maintain that lean muscle and keep it functioning. In short, the more muscle you have, the more calories you can consume without gaining any additional body fat. Muscle turns your body into a fat-burning machine, and who doesn't love that idea?

EXERCISE DENSITY

"Exercise density" is simply the amount of work you will perform in any given amount of time. My goal is to have you work harder and more effectively in a shorter time frame. The goal of HIIT is to make the most of your time—in most cases, twenty to thirty minutes or less. By increasing your intensity and decreasing your training time, you optimize your muscular activity and cardiovascular endurance. This is critical in both cardio health and sports performance. With HIIT you are getting the most work done in the shortest amount of time, minimizing impact on joints, and reducing potential overuse injuries, all while giving your body the ultimate potential for results.

HOW DO I START?

So here's the deal: high-intensity training is *intense!* Lots of people jump in unprepared and they end up injured because their sudden motivation didn't match their physical ability. When starting out, one to two HIIT sessions are enough for the first few weeks.

A few rules to live by if you choose to do HIIT:

- **Always put safety first**—Be smart. Don't overdo your workouts thinking it will lead you to success faster. You will only end up hurt and back at square one with potential burnout or, worse, injury. When you increase weight keep it reasonable: an increase of 5 percent or less from the maximum weight you lifted the last time you did the same exercise. Keeping a training log can help you keep track. Continue to add load as you become stronger.

- **Don't skip the warm-up**—A dynamic warm-up, such as mountain climbers, jumping jacks, jump roping, or jogging, will activate and prepare your entire body for the training ahead as well as increase your core and muscle temperature. Aim for five to ten minutes for your warm-up.

- **Choose your weights wisely**—A pretty basic rule of thumb when picking weights is to choose a weight that will allow you to complete the suggested number of repetitions with perfect form while feeling fatigued by the end of the rep. This is how you break down your muscles so they can grow back stronger after rest and recovery.

- **Remember your form is critical**—I see so many people who compromise their form in order to lift heavier weights. At all times your form should be excellent or you are adding too much load. As a general rule, back straight, spine neutral, and knees slightly bent. If you have to swing the weights to complete the rep, you need to drop the load.

- **Make a great effort**—Again, safety and form come first, but remember, this is meant to be *intense,* so don't expect to be able to carry on a long conversation or pick up a magazine and read in the middle of a workout. Give it your maximum effort, and you will get excellent results.

- **Remember to recover**—What happens outside the gym is just as critical, if not more, as what happens inside the gym. If you want to get the very most out of your training remember to recover with solid rest. Aim for seven to nine hours of sleep each night and one to two rest days a week (minimum) to enable your body to repair and grow stronger. Also, don't forget that food is the biggest part of the fat loss equation, so if you don't eat for success the work you do in the gym won't show.

Homework: Force Field Analysis

When I was a little girl my father made me complete a simple task every time I had a difficult decision. This task has stuck with me my entire life, and I have used it during some of my toughest choices, from which city to live in to which university I should attend (Go Blue!) even to whether to leave a job and become a fitness coach (my best choice ever). Now I'm going to share his task with all of you. I hope it helps to lend the same clarity.

For your homework this week, I want you to think about how you might be numbing your pain after your loss. Are you having that nightly glass of wine that turns into two or three? Are you relying on unhealthy food, controlled substances, or avoidance behavior? Think about how this is negatively affecting your life.

Next, do a force field analysis of what you might be using as avoidance behavior. What is a force field analysis? My dad will be thrilled you asked. Take a blank piece of paper and write your numbing behavior at the top (if you have more than one numbing behavior, use more than one sheet of paper). Below the numbing behavior make two columns, a pro column and a con column. Now list the pros and cons of your behavior, and be honest. Even if you're using something to numb your pain, it doesn't have to be all negative, so don't skip this process. Really think through your two columns and consider sleeping on them throughout the week. By the end of this week I hope you have an honest and realistic viewpoint of your behavior and how it is playing into other areas of your life. Is social drinking keeping you from waking up earlier and going after your goals? Is eating more sweets making you irritable and cranky with your friends and family? If you see your behavior laid out in black and white, you are more likely to face it and decide if it benefits your life going forward. If it does not, work to drop it and move in a more positive and life-affirming direction. If you wish, share your force field analysis with your Healthy Healing online community.

Planning for the Future

About a year after the death of my husband I decided to quit my corporate job and follow my dream of helping the world see fitness as a grief-coping mechanism. It was a scary and bold move and one that was not readily accepted by everyone who knew and loved me. In my heart I knew it was my only choice, and I felt a deep and residing peace around my decision. The money didn't matter, and for the first time in my life I realized I couldn't wait any longer to make my dreams come true. Life was too short. It took death and widowhood for me to see what needed to be done, but it was crystal clear to me finally.

Why do we put off the things we really want to do in life till a day in the distant future? Do we really think we have endless days to make our dreams a reality? I think before we experience death we do believe that bad things happen to other people and we have all the time in the world to make our lives count. We waste time like it's replaceable, and we don't think twice about the time we give to others, saying yes to things we'd rather say no to. Death makes us reevaluate

Week 9 Baby Steps

FITNESS:

_____

_____

_____

NUTRITION:

_____

_____

_____

HAPPINESS:

_____

_____

_____

PERSONAL GROWTH:

_____

_____

_____

how we spend our time and why we make choices that often don't lead us to our best life. Death reminds us, in no uncertain terms, of what we put off in the past and makes us face the regrets we have in the present.

If you could do it all again, what would you do differently? What would you plan and how big would you decide to live? You can't go back and change what happened in your past, but you have the choice right now to make the most of what comes next. This week I want you to think about what you have been putting off. Is there something you want to do or something that would help you move forward but you feel like you should wait? This week will be all about letting go of what's holding you back, allowing yourself to envision what your new future will look like, and how you can live the life you've always wanted, even if it's different than you imagined.

Choosing to Live Again

One of the things death has taught me is that we make time for what is important to us, but sometimes, especially when things really matter, we still put them off for another day. I remember that Mitch and I talked about hiking the Kalalau Trail on the Na Pali Coast of Kauai, but we kept putting it off, year after year, because we believed we had time. We never made it a priority. It was always "next year" and then we had babies and next year turned into "when the kids are bigger." We never did it. We ran out of time and he never got to take that hike because death had other plans. After his death, I vowed to put the hike and so many of our other dreams on my calendar and make them happen in his honor. Finally, in May of 2014, I did that hike; it now serves as one of my life's greatest memories. I remember coming to mile four of the trail and standing on a hill that overlooked the entire valley. It was the most beautiful shade of green I had ever seen—waterfalls in every direction and the dark volcanic rock peeking through the lush rain forest walls. Tears filled up my eyes, and I said, "It's so beautiful, it almost does not even look real. Oh my goodness, he would have loved this." Those moments are ripe with duality—so much joy for living his dream, regardless of how painful it was, and yet so much sorrow that he was not there to live that dream himself. It was a magical hike that left me feeling inspired to do and see more without wasting precious time. Two days after the hike I decided to also kayak the coast for good measure, knowing he'd approve of my ambitious tenacity. The coast has been called the Everest of sea kayaking, so I was nervous, but this too now serves as a great memory of my life. Seeing Na Pali from that vantage point as well was abundantly and spiritually healing for my soul. I wouldn't trade those few days of my life for anything. Knowing I lived his list and honored my life after the loss of him has given me moments I will always be thankful for.

The truth is, you won't ever have enough time for anything if you don't make a plan and make it happen. You have to put it on the calendar, make it a priority, save the money, and complete the dream. Yes, it really is that simple. Maybe money is a concern, so you put the item down for a year from now. Maybe during the next year you cut out your daily coffee stop. Maybe you take a side job or stop buying endless junk from the mall. I decided a long time ago that I was going to stop being a "consumer" unless it was something that was truly a "need" and not something that would be in and out of my house within a two-week period. That helps me focus on the bigger goals of my life and avoid buying useless junk. At the end of the day, you can live on purpose and make it happen or you can live with excuses and regret. The choice is up to you.

Purging and Letting Go

Loss teaches us many lessons. Some of these lessons are big and significant: Don't sweat the small stuff. Make sure to tell the people you love that they are important while they are alive. Some of our lessons are smaller, less significant, but equally as valuable to the quality of the lives we lead. One of the greatest lessons I've taken from loss is that less is more. Letting go of material possessions has helped me feel more alive, more present, and more free. I've found that the more I let go, the lighter and happier I feel.

I will never forget the thoughts that obsessed me during the first twenty-four hours after my loss. When your loss comes as a shock, your brain does strange things you'd never expect and never be able to plan for. My brain kept taking a mental stock of everything valuable in my life that still mattered. Of course, my children topped my list, as did my friends and family, who came rushing to my side that dreadful day. The only other measurable thing I could think of that mattered was all the memories I had created with my late husband. It was as if my own life was flashing before my eyes, and what mattered most were the things we had done, the memories we had created, and the adventures we had lived. Nothing material even entered the equation. I didn't think about our house, our cars, our furniture, or even our bank account. In fact, I didn't inventory anything material at all. Loss reveals the true value of life, and to me that value was not in anything that could be bought or owned. Now, I've never been much of a material person; however, my revelation was interesting, even to me. All of the clichés that remind us "You can't take it with you" came rushing to mind as life's greatest truths.

Yes, less is more, but letting go of material things that belonged to the person we loved is not an easy process. We hold on to material items hoping that the memories they provide can help us retain parts of them. I kept Mitch's deodorant for years, just so I could take off the cap and smell it when I needed to feel him close. For the first year, I hardly touched his side of the bathroom or his closet. I hardly touched anything of his unless I slept in one of his shirts or cleaned a picture frame. Several months after, I collected a box of his favorite clothing and mailed it to my sister, who kindly offered to make quilts out of his things for me and the kids. As I collected the items that would go into the box, I realized just how hard the process of purging and letting go was going to be, and as I placed each item into the box, I felt like I was saying good-bye over and over again. As I keep reminding you, loss is not a linear, neat process that follows a well-defined path. Loss is messy, awkward, bumpy, and confusing, never taking a straight road and never what you expect it to be. Many people think that the loss itself is the hardest part, but truthfully the loss is just the beginning. As we collect their things, purge their life, and move forward with our unplanned future, we grieve in a million new ways every single day. It's a daunting and exhausting process that tires the soul. But eventually letting go brings some inner peace.

In your own time, you will feel the strength and the need to let go of more stuff. You will start to find that all the extra things in your life are nothing more than added weight, that the person you lost remains with you in memories, thoughts, and stories. There is nothing that will tell you the right time to purge, but you will start to feel the weight in your life and begin to crave a simpler, cleaner, and more deliberate future. Start small and be willing to walk away when the emotional toll becomes too great. Start with a box or a bag, and when you are done, congratulate yourself on the steps you took. Day after day, week after week, year after year, you will let go. You will remember that feeling you had after loss and that your love lies not in the stuff you've kept but in the freedom from stuff. The ability to really live is what will help you create a new life as you move forward.

Purging the Pantry

So far in this book I've asked you to take numerous small baby steps toward a better life, but now I'm going to have you take a bigger step. I want you to purge your pantry of anything that is not benefiting your body and your new lifestyle. I still want you to live an 80/20 lifestyle, but the 20 percent does not have to be staring you in the face every single day, testing your willpower. Instead, save the 20 percent for when you are eating out or simply outside your home, and keep your home a place that supports your goals for a better, more nutritious life.

Letting Go of Preconceived Expectations

Our society has many antiquated rules that, in my opinion, harm our growth as individuals. Vishen Lakhiani, founder of Mindvalley, talks about this at great length in his book *The Code of the Extraordinary Mind*—a book I strongly recommended because many of his principles can be applied to grief. He talks about the "brules," as he calls them—the bullshit rules that are the day-to-day norms we all follow, without questioning their usefulness to our well-being.[1] We have rules in every aspect of our lives, ranging from how we parent to how we educate ourselves and our children to of course how we face grief. I've already told you my thoughts about the "grief box" and not trying to conform to how society tells you to successfully grieve, but what about fitness? Are there preconceived rules around fitness that you blindly follow? Think about how many times you decided to go to the gym to "work off" a meal you ate the night before. Have you done a particular kind of exercise because you've been conditioned to think you must do that exercise in order to be successfully fit? Your view of fitness has been largely shaped by outside forces and passed down from generations that came before. It's time for you to let all that go and understand that you can be successful with your fitness if you do *anything* consistently. Similarly, you may need to let go of preconceived notions about what a healthy body looks like. You've probably been conditioned to believe that skinny is healthy when in reality it can be very unhealthy. It's time to let go of all that too and instead aim to be strong, fit, and alive. I want you to live your one fit life fully and completely and far away from society's brules.

Homework: Vision Boards

Six months after Mitch died, I took my children to Sedona for the day with some friends. It was our way of "celebrating" the day because Mitch loved Sedona. It was one of his favorite places to fly, lost among the red rocks, taking in the grand beauty of the desert. We had a pretty nice day, just my best girlfriends and our kids. Being with my friends, without their husbands, always made me feel a little less alone, so the day went by without an overload of pain, until later that evening when one of them posted a photo on Facebook of me and my two kids. In that moment I saw the triangle. We had gone from being a family of four to a family of three, and the triangle made me feel sad for our future.

So here you are, facing your new normal, wishing for the life you had before and wondering how you'll start creating the life that will be. Moving forward takes strength and fortitude, but that's why you're doing the work in this book. This week's homework is meant to help you start to think about the future you'd like to create beyond loss. I understand moving forward may be hard to face, but it is a necessary step in the process of being an active participant in your grief. One of the things you lost when your loved one died was the future you wanted to create with that person. Perhaps you feel like you lost yourself as well. When your person died so did the person you were before your loss. When your person died so did the future you'd planned around their presence.

This week's baby step will be to create a vision board. Vision boards are valuable tools to focus you on the positive things you'd like to create for your life. They can help you achieve goals and create forward movement. There are many ways to create a vision board. You can do it the old-fashioned way and cut out photos from magazines that you place on a large board you keep somewhere in your home. The benefit to creating a physical board is that you will see it daily and be reminded of your goals and intentions for the future. Wherever you decide to place it, it should be somewhere you visit often, to inspire you to keep moving forward on a daily basis. If that seems like too much work and you'd rather make a virtual board, there are numerous free apps to help you create fun boards from photos you store online— PicMonkey, PicCollage, and Collage Maker, to name a few. These apps allow you to drop and drag in photos and give you plenty of spaces to fill up with your new dreams. What you place on your board is entirely up to you. I'd suggest that you keep your board varied and fill it with fitness inspiration, healthy living, travel, bucket lists, family, or whatever makes you feel alive and inspired. Also include what you'd like to focus on for the next part of your life. As you sit and look at the photos you've collected you may feel overwhelmed. Remember that regardless of what you've been through, you can shape the future in a positive way. And you don't have to make these changes all at once! The purpose of this homework is to give you a road map as you begin your steps forward.

Leading by Example

I remember the first time someone called me "strong" after Mitch's death. It happened the day after his death, and believe me I was not strong in that moment. In fact, I was particularly dead inside. I remember the words made me feel so sad because I wasn't really being strong as much as I was just surviving. I was doing what I had to do, as hard as each day was. The truth is, if you are making a conscious effort to improve your life after your loss, you are strong. The easiest choice you can make is to give up, bide your time, and let life pass you by. So by not giving up you are making a harder choice today that will improve your life tomorrow. By making this difficult choice you are likely inspiring the world around you, even if that's not your motivation. You are causing a positive ripple whether you see it or not, and you are reminding others that they too can do hard things. I don't want you to own that responsibility. It can become daunting to be everyone's inspiration, and you shouldn't feel the need to inspire others at all. But I do want you to recognize your amazing inner spirit. You are surviving, even on days when you are hardly breathing. That is incredible. Don't forget to give yourself credit for all that you are and how you're surviving what most people can't even fathom.

Week 10 Baby Steps

FITNESS:

_____

_____

_____

NUTRITION:

_____

_____

_____

HAPPINESS:

_____

_____

_____

PERSONAL GROWTH:

_____

_____

_____

This week you'll learn how to keep yourself and the people around you healthy. We'll talk about how to stay fit on a budget, when to choose organic and non-organic foods, and then tackle perhaps my favorite homework assignment in the entire book.

Show the Way

Empowering you to live a full and fit life is one of my greatest goals with this book. As much as I want to give you that gift with all my heart and soul, you have to go out and do it for yourself. I can preach, lecture, nag, and beg, but only you can make it happen.

When I discovered the power of this healing process, I wanted to share it with my kids. I remember when I'd tell my then three-year-old daughter that Mommy was going to the gym she'd say, "Mommy is going to get *strong!!*" and we'd both laugh. She was so right. I was going to strengthen my mind, body, and spirit.

When she was a little older, I signed her up for the Iron Girl race in Arizona. Iron Girl is an event held around the country that enables moms and daughters to run a race together as a way to encourage fitness and bonding. This race was a 5K run, and at the time we signed up, three-plus miles seemed like a big goal for my six-year-old girl. I asked Addison if she wanted to run with her mommy, and she ecstatically said, "*Yes!*" I think she wanted to spend time with me, doing something she knew I loved, but I also think all my running had inspired her to give it a try. I've done countless races and I know, firsthand, just how powerful they can be. I couldn't wait to share that feeling and make that memory with her at such an early age. Race morning came, and I will never forget how excited we both were. It was my birthday that day, and I couldn't imagine a better way to have spent it. We got up early and headed to the course in Fountain Hills, Arizona. Addison was nervous, but we got signed in, grabbed our race bibs, and made our way to the starting corral. As we stood there waiting for the race to start, I could see the excitement in her eyes. The music was blaring, the energy was electric, and my daughter's face was overcome with happiness. She looked over at me and said, "Mommy, this is awesome," and I just knew she was hooked. We started the race full of energy, and the crowd cheered us on as we went. She ran hard, the crowd pushing us on and the adrenaline giving her strength. About halfway through her little legs started to get tired, and she looked over at me and asked if I could carry her. As hard as it was on me as her mom, I told her, no, I could not. I told her she had to finish the race by herself in order for it to count. We slowed down and shifted between a walk and a slow jog. As she put one foot in front of the other, on her own, the struggle she was pushing through was having a far greater impact than if I had made it easy. We walked, then ran, then walked some more until we finally sprinted across the finish line together. As we crossed over the line, I heard my daughter's name said over the loudspeaker, congratulating her on being an "Iron Girl." You could not wipe the smile off her little face. She was so proud of what she had just done, and it gave her an undeniable bout of self-confidence, self-worth, and validation.

I see this as a coach as well, and I see it in all areas of my clients' lives. Difficult moments, coupled with the strength to keep going, elevate our inner strength. As I'm helping my clients never give up, they are helping themselves to a better life. The road will not be easy, your legs will get tired, but you must never quit. I always ask my clients "What are you going to do when you quit? Quit and do what?" Will you simply stop, fall back into negative habits, become more miserable, and then start again in six months, further back from where you started originally? Even if you can't move forward for a while, don't give up! Take a break, rest your mind, your body, and/or your spirit—whatever needs the most rest—and begin again. At least you didn't quit.

People ask me all the time how they can change the health habits of the people around them. I always laugh and come back with the same response: "Lead by example." You can't force the people you love to exercise, to eat right, or to live a fit lifestyle. You can't force them to try to heal from their losses in a healthy and productive manner. Regardless of how much wisdom you impart, no matter how many stats you throw their way, the people you love are only going to do what they are ready to do. When they hit their own rock bottom they will change and not a moment before. Motivation does not last, inspiration comes and goes, and change is often fleeting, but when someone sits near the bottom of their existence and realizes that they alone are responsible for their happiness and they alone can change their life, that change will stick.

While you can't make someone change, you can be a positive influence on how they perceive a fit lifestyle. Most people believe that being fit is all about deprivation. What I try to teach people is that living a fit life is all about having more of the best that life offers. That when your body feels good because you've been eating foods that make you thrive, and when your body is strong and capable of accomplishing any goal you set out for it, you can live with much more purpose than you ever imagined. Fitness is not about giving up a good life; fitness is about gaining the best life.

You can't force anyone to see the value in fitness, but you can show them. The very best way to positively affect the people around you is to lead by example. Show them why fitness matters. Show them why whole foods matter. Most of all, show them why *you* matter, and they just might start to envision a similar path for themselves. Leading by example also empowers you in knowing that you make a difference.

Giving back and helping others is one of the greatest is the roads to healthy healing. When you start a ripple effect that shapes the world around you in a better way you heal another small corner of your own heart.

Healthy on a Budget

I hear it again and again: eating healthy is cost prohibitive. The cost associated with health intimidates many of us and can cause failure before a fair chance is given to forming new healthy habits. Eating healthy can be expensive if you don't plan or you waste food, but in my experience, once you figure out your food portions, eating well is actually cheaper than eating poorly. Before I talk more about budget, I want to remind you what you are gaining with a whole-foods lifestyle. You are potentially avoiding preventable diseases. You are building your immunity and allowing your cells to heal your body, therefore avoiding medical bills and lost productivity down the road. Food may not guarantee a perfectly healthy future, but it sure does tip the scales in the right direction. This especially frustrates me when it comes to our kids. We won't spare any expense getting them the best sports equipment, coaches, teachers, and stylish clothing, but when it comes to their food, we go cheap. Invest in your health and invest in the health of the people you love, because at the end of the day it matters more than any high-priced coach ever could.

The following list of tips comes in part from my sister, Lorrie McFadden, who is the certified nutrition consultant for My1FitLife. Lorrie came to the world of nutrition, like so many others, looking for a way to feel better after years of making poor food choices, struggling with weight issues, and noticing the impact poor food choices were having on her overall health. Lorrie worked with My1FitLife as a client and found the changes so profound she discovered nutrition as a life's calling, and she continued her personal education in this field and eventually joined our team. Below she reminds us eating clean is becoming more affordable every day.

Tips for Saving Money[1]

Here's a list of easy ways to save money when grocery shopping:

- Shop close to home to avoid hassle and added gas expense. Big-box stores like Costco have good products, often at deep discounts. Don't be afraid of bulk buying; just be prepared to appropriately freeze what can't be consumed quickly. For example, I buy organic spinach in bulk from Costco, and I wash, dry, and freeze what I can't use for my morning smoothie. I also have a Costco list that is separate from what I buy at my regular grocer or a specialty store like Trader Joe's. I typically shop when I'm closest to each store, and I keep a running list of what I need.

- Take coupons when you can or look for savings apps from your local stores. Remain flexible with your purchases so you can get the best deals.

- Shop in season and freeze ahead of time. I live in a state where many fruits and vegetables have to be shipped in over large distances, which ends up driving up the prices and diminishing the foods' nutrient levels. Buy what is in season and locally grown, and plan ahead during your summer months with good storage methods in mind (freezing or canning).

- Prepare meals in large batches. This not only saves you time but also provides additional meals, and most products are cheaper when purchased in bulk.

- Get to know your grocer. Don't be afraid to befriend the store manager and ask about special product ordering. The more your store hears about its community's interest in clean eating, the more organic food the store will stock on its shelves and the more interest will grow, hopefully bringing prices down. Don't be afraid to make your voice heard.

- Whenever possible, don't buy precut foods. You are paying for someone else's labor. Take the prep time we talked about earlier and do it yourself.

- Join a local CSA (community-supported agriculture) or organic food group. They are popping up all over, and they can help you save money as well as provide you with fresh, farm-to-table goodness.

- Avoid packaged foods. These foods are not as healthy and there is added expense for materials and time. Not to mention the wear on our environment and resources. Spend more of your budget at local farmers' markets, most of whose venders bring their food straight to you from the earth.

- Consider purchasing BPA-free storage containers, which can be found at local stores or online. Rather than buying canned foods, freeze chicken broth, sauces, greens for your smoothies, leftovers, and extra foods from your garden. Use your storage system to house a pretty pantry full of bulk items, such as flour, beans, granola, and rice. It is far less expensive to buy bulk rice than to buy a microwave version, a precooked frozen bag, or a premixed blend.

- Host a cooking meet-up. This is a great way to add in community, get new recipe ideas, and have some fun. Together you can make large batches of chili, soups, sauces, healthy cookies, and salad dressings. Divvy them up and save. You can take turns offering up your kitchen while others buy the groceries, and you split the costs.

- Grow your own. Okay, I know that's a big request and very time-consuming, but it just may become therapeutic and limit your stress. Growing greens and herbs is a simple way to start. If you have limited space, grow a few items in pots. You can also grow eight to ten varieties of greens most of the year with just an 8-foot-square plot that gets some sun. You can also grow herbs on a sunny indoor windowsill or tomatoes on your patio.

Organic vs. Non-Organic

There are credible reasons behind the recent organic push in the world. Pesticides cover our foods, and today's overworked agricultural soil is often missing the vital nutrients our bodies need to repair and regrow. While I think buying organic is important, I'm not going to ask you to eat 100 percent organic foods. But it does help if you learn where not to cut corners.

The following list of produce, based on the Environmental Working Group's "Dirty Dozen,"[2] includes the conventionally grown fruits and vegetables notorious for being highly toxic and testing positive for roughly fifty chemicals. For these items, *go organic*! It's worth the extra dollars.

Apples	Grapes
Celery	Hot peppers
Cherries	Nectarines

Peaches	Strawberries
Pears	Sweet bell peppers
Potatoes	Tomatoes
Spinach	

On the other hand, these "Clean 15" (also based on the Environmental Working Group's list) are typically lower in toxins and chemicals, even grown conventionally, and they can be bought at most grocery stores.[3]

Asparagus	Honeydew melon
Avocados	Kiwi
Cabbage	Mangos
Cantaloupe	Onions
Cauliflower	Papayas
Eggplant	Pineapples
Grapefruit	Sweet peas, frozen

My rule of thumb is if it has a peel that will be discarded—like a banana, grapefruit, or watermelon—I feel okay about buying non-organic. If I will eat the fruit or vegetable whole—like apples, berries, greens, or grapes—I go organic.

Overuse Injuries

As fitness becomes a bigger part of your life, it is important to take care of your body and its joints, tendons, ligaments, and muscles. When I first started my fitness journey I had a tendency to overdo it.

I beat down my body, not thinking about the long-term ramifications of the damage I was doing. Exercise is a wonderful thing, and fitness is a positive for your life, but just like anything else, it can be overdone.

Overuse injuries most often occur when the same muscle groups, joints, ligaments, or tendons are used to the point of damage. This can happen when you train the same way for long periods of time without mixing up your routine. For example, runners can become prone to knee problems from the repetitive pounding, and lifters can see shoulder injuries thanks to impingement of the shoulder capsule (the ligaments surrounding the joint) or lifting heavy weights for too long. The key is to vary your workouts so you can avoid fatigued muscles that end up causing you long-term issues. For example, in the workout programs I put together for my clients, I never have the client do the same thing multiple weeks in a row. The program will have higher intensity cardio weeks followed by weeks of higher reps and lower weights, then periods of higher weights and lower reps followed by a week or two of a "deloading" phase. Deloading is when you purposefully tone down your training in order to allow for repair and regrowth. Within the fitness world this is all controversial, and depending on who you ask you will get ten different answers about it, but the key is to listen to your body and make sure you avoid stressing the same muscles in the same way week after week. Variety is the spice of life, and that goes for your workouts as well. In addition to preventing injuries, it will help you avoid plateaus. Keeping your workouts fresh is always a good thing.

Homework: Living Like a Fit Person

I've been a stressed out, overworked person determined to put everything and everyone before myself because I somehow figured it made me a better wife, mom, employee, or friend. I've also been a fit person who takes the time for me, prioritizes my health and fitness, and doesn't make excuses for doing it! What I discovered through my personal life experimentation is that by putting even a nominal effort into my health and fitness I actually became a better wife, mom, employee, and friend. For true change, you will have to start with your mindset. When you change your mindset and shift your priorities, not only will your body change but, more importantly, your life will change as well. It won't matter what anyone around you thinks of your new lifestyle if you believe in its value at your core.

You can choose to not exercise, not move your body, not eat well, and not surround yourself with a positive and uplifting community, or you can choose to move each day a little more, pick exercises you love to do, add more nutritious foods to your diet, and surround yourself with the kind of people who make your life better. The beautiful thing about life is that you have the choice, and your choices will define how you spend much of your future.

This week's homework is truly one of my personal favorites for many reasons. I call this "LLAFP," which is short for Living Like a Fit Person. I believe that fitness—both physical and mental—is a choice that takes time and requires patience. With this challenge I want you to make the conscious and deliberate choice to LLAFP every single day for the next week. No, that does not mean I want you to work out every single day, because rest is very important to your fitness, your body's development, and your overall health, but I do want you to see the simple, easy ways you can LLAFP for the rest of your life, every single day, starting right now. This homework isn't about big leaps and bounds but small, deliberate steps in the right direction.

During this week I also want you to take a photo of yourself each day while doing something that makes you healthier, happier, and ultimately more fit. Maybe you park farther from the grocery store and walk in. Maybe you take the stairs at work or at the airport. Maybe you pick veggies at lunch over the french fries. Maybe you work your butt off in the gym, or maybe you go for a beautiful hike in nature. I don't care what it is, but I do care that you make the choice to live healthy and with intention. If you'd like, share your photos online with the hashtag #healthyhealing or post them with the program's community via the online portal. We want to know that you are kicking butt and doing the homework so we can cheer you on. The purpose of the photos is to remind you that you are making this choice daily and your choices make you. You can also create a collage of your seven days to help congratulate yourself and give you motivation as you move forward. Go you!

Living in the Moment

Modern society has told us that we need to have a good education, a fancy job, a nice car, and a big house to be happy and successful. We are told that success, and therefore happiness, is a measurable commodity that exists within a framework of stability. When one day you wake up and find that someone close to you is now gone, throwing that framework into an unstable spin, you begin to question everything you were ever told and have ever learned. This may be the very first time in your life that you don't blindly accept the status quo. You may start to imagine a life that looks completely different from the life you have been living.

This happened to me after my loss, and it hit me with a huge bang! I had the dream job with a fancy title and a secure paycheck, but it all seemed so empty after Mitch died. My gut told me I should teach fitness as a grief-coping mechanism, but I didn't know how and I was scared to leave my secure job. Until one day, shortly after I had returned to work after Mitch died, my boss told me that a client wanted to speak with me. My job, as head of real estate for a private destination club, entailed securing multimillion-dollar properties for

Week 11 Baby Steps

FITNESS:

_____

_____

_____

NUTRITION:

_____

_____

_____

HAPPINESS:

_____

_____

_____

PERSONAL GROWTH:

_____

_____

_____

very wealthy clients around the world. My boss informed me that we had an unhappy guest staying at one of our exquisite properties in Mexico, and he wanted to speak with someone in the acquisitions department. I got on the phone with this man and listened to him complain about the three-million-dollar home he was staying in because the negative-edge pool at the house, the one with a view of both the Sea of Cortez *and* the Pacific Ocean, was not nearly big enough. It took everything in my power not to tell the guy to screw off and hang up on him. I quit my job shortly after to fulfill my gut instinct, which led me to writing this book for all of you.

Perspective changes with death, and what society considers important may no longer match your viewpoint. This new perspective is one of the gifts of grief, and this week's focus will help you harness the unique perspective you now have and explore the concept of really living again after loss.

I was hard on Mitch pretty often and for things that I regret today. I remember relentlessly making him miserable because I wanted him to be more driven, to want a bigger house, a nicer car, and a fatter bank account. I wanted him to wake up one morning and strive to be very successful, to win the big job, and to give us a beautiful life. I'd often ask him "Where do you want to be in five years?" and his prophetic response would always be "We don't know if we will be here in five years, so why does it matter?" He'd tell me to "live in the moment," and I'd laugh and think that he was simpleminded. In fact, in our fifteen years together, I always assumed that I had been put on this earth to teach him grand lessons on life. I was sure that I was here to show him how to want more, be more, and achieve more.

Mitch was self-actualized in so many ways, and he had a spirit of joy, happiness, and peace. He never wanted for more and always was content with what he had. There is a beauty to that awareness and a high form of existence. I didn't recognize his evolution until it was too late, when I realized that I was the one with the lower form of human consciousness. In his death, I realized that instead of me being the teacher, Mitch had been the one doing the teaching all along. His lesson of "living in the moment" was the one I most desperately needed to learn, and in many ways still do.

Even today, all these years later, I still struggle with the concept of living in the moment. I think we all do. We constantly want more, strive for bigger, and think we need better. The problem is that "more," "bigger," and "better" are often linked to monetary possessions or temporary states of being. We find momentary happiness or joy in something we buy, a song we hear, or a meal we eat. Once the new-car smell wears off, the song stops playing, or the meal is done, we find ourselves searching for that next "thing" that will make us happy. Instead, we should be searching for internal happiness that can't be heightened or dampened by outside forces.

Living in the moment takes daily practice and is much easier said than done. I've found that my daily five- to ten-minute meditation practice has helped me focus more on the now and less on what was or what might be. Living in the moment is about gaining control over your mind and your thoughts, and mediation is a powerful way to increase mental control and clarity. I often practice enjoying my present state regardless of my activity. If only for a few moments, I make myself focus on the now and take stock of my current level of gratitude and thankfulness. I haven't mastered this concept yet, but it's one I continue to work on all the time. From enjoying family time while cooking to having the chance to reflect and read the words in this book, each moment is a gift. We waste that gift when we worry about what's not there or what we can't control instead of appreciating what is and what we can do.

Eating New Foods

When was the last time you tried something new in the kitchen? We get stuck in a rut, especially after loss, because we tend to take the path of least resistance. It's human nature to take the easiest and quickest road, but one of my goals in this book it to get you out of all kinds of ruts, from fitness to nutrition to grief. I keep my kitchen out of a rut by making one new meal a week—talk about baby steps! I don't promise myself that I will create a new masterpiece several days a week; instead, I pick one day—typically Sunday—find a recipe online that looks good, and prepare it as a test to see if it makes it into the rotation. By picking only one day for this, I look forward to preparing something new without the daunting thought of doing it several times a week.

This week I'd like you to do this too. Pick one new dish and give it a try. Choose from the recipes later in the book (page 251) or find other options on the program's website (www.healthyhealingbook .com/healing), where there is also a list of some of my favorite blogs for additional great healthy recipes!

Trying Something New

It's easy to get comfortable with your fitness choices too, and as we've discussed, this can lead to plateaus and overuse injuries. This week I'd like you to try one new form of fitness and see how it "fits" with your personality. Maybe it's a Zumba class at the gym, a boot camp group, or even something empowering like Krav Maga (Israeli fighting). The key is to keep mixing it up and finding new things you love to do to keep you inspired and moving forward. When you find something new you love, incorporate it into your routine and consider yourself one of the lucky few who truly understands the value of fitness and what it adds to your life. With each new discipline you have a new stress-coping tool to add to your grief toolbox. With anything new you've found, make sure you hashtag #healthyhealing on your social networks and online at the program's interactive portal.

Homework: Bucket List

On the night Mitch died, I thought I was done. With his death, everything we had ever dreamed of doing as a couple and with our kids was now lost. I thought I couldn't possibly do it by myself. His crash was my own personal death sentence. I felt so weak, so tired, and so incredibly lost without him. It's a uniquely lonely feeling when you've lived and loved so much and it all falls away in a split second.

As I leaned on fitness in those early days, I started to feel a small fire burn after every workout. The sweat gave me a clarity of mind and a strength of spirit that seemed all but lost in my moments of stillness. I'd finish a workout and hear my inner voice start to whisper, *You can still live.* I'd squelch the voice and return to my defeatist mindset until the next workout, when the voice spoke a little louder: *Michelle, you can still live . . . I want you to live.* The thought of living fully took my breath away, and every emotion—from guilt to anger to fear—rose up within me. Finally, after a few weeks, the voice was so loud I couldn't ignore it any longer. I grabbed a piece of paper and began to write. I wrote tirelessly for the next few hours. I wrote every wish and dream that Mitch had ever had, that I had ever had, and that we had had for ourselves as a couple and as the parents of Addison and Matthew. As I wrote, I reminded myself that Mitch had loved life, had loved adventure, and had loved to travel. It had been so important to him that we do the things that made us feel alive and, as our kids grew, show them the meaning of living a full life. I was resolved for the first time since his passing to teach my kids who he had been by showing them how he had lived.

Shortly after that, I started to take every day that should've been sad and difficult and turn it into a day when I honored Mitch. By living his list, my list, and our list, I live a life he would have wanted me to live. I've hiked fourteeners in Colorado (peaks of at least 14,000 feet!) and ocean-side cliffs in Kauai. I've rafted rivers he had wanted to run with rapids as exhilarating as any on earth. I've traveled to far-off countries, run a marathon, and moved to the mountains. I've also taken our kids to their first day of kindergarten and started a nonprofit in his honor.

I've repeatedly told you to take baby steps to your goals—I never want you to feel like you have to leap—but at this moment I want to remind you that if you don't dream big, you will never do anything big. You can still use the concept of baby steps to reach your goals, but ideally I'd like you to aim high when you consider this week's homework. As a general rule, we tend to underestimate what we can do, so think bigger than you would typically for your bucket list.

Your big dreams and big goals may look nothing like mine. You may wish to go back to school rather than raft a river. You may dream of playing a musical instrument, learning a foreign language, or seeing a long-lost relative. It's time to dream big. Write down your pie-in-the-sky dreams and start taking those baby steps to make them happen.

These goals may seem out of reach but you can do them because you've already lived through so much worse. A friend once told me very early on after my loss, "Once you bury your husband, you can do anything." How true is that? It also has helped me to remember how much Mitch loved me. I fulfilled that list of goals for him until I found the strength to do it for myself. The person you lost loved you too.

On the following page, fill in your bucket list—or life list, list of intentions, whatever you wish to call it. Once you have done that, choose one item you can realistically make happen this year and two more that you can make happen within the next three years. Give this some good thought and make sure you are honest with yourself about what you can accomplish. After narrowing down your list, put the three items on your calendar and the date you wish to have them accomplished by. Schedule check-in dates too, to hold yourself accountable for your goals. I encourage you to transform any harder-than-hard days from something painful into something beautiful. For example, when I'm standing on top of a mountain on the anniversary of Mitch's death, it turns a day that could be tragic and sad into a day full of possibility and hope. Finally, post your list on the program's online portal and hashtag #healthyhealing on social media.

If you are a widowed person who needs some financial support to achieve a bucket-list dream, you can also apply for sponsorship through our Live the List nonprofit (www.livethelistnonprofit.org).

Bucket List

_____

_____

_____

_____

_____

_____

_____

_____

_____

_____

_____

_____

_____

_____

_____

_____

_____

Honoring the Person You Lost

It's hard to believe we are at Week 12 already. While this is the end of my weekly instruction, it is just the beginning of your new, empowered, fit life. Everything you have learned so far can be repeated as necessary. Continue to work through the program again and again, because each time you will learn something new about yourself, your body, and your life. I've had people take my online twelve-week program for a year straight and tell me that each time they learned a different lesson and made new positive choices. Don't expect to be an expert after twelve weeks; just commit to those baby steps and continue moving forward. I'm so proud of the work you've done and will continue to do for your best life! In this final week your focus will be on moving forward while honoring, healing, and releasing in the healthiest ways.

One way I've felt really peaceful about my steps forward after my loss is to look at my accomplishments as a form of honoring Mitch. Many of my races have been dedicated to his memory. There is something about running in honor of that person you lost and will always love. They aren't with you, but they're there in spirit when you cross

Week 12 Baby Steps

FITNESS:

_____

_____

_____

NUTRITION:

_____

_____

_____

HAPPINESS:

_____

_____

_____

PERSONAL GROWTH:

_____

_____

_____

the finish line, and the meaning you give to the run makes it cleansing and cathartic. You may feel joy, sorrow, anger, and pride, all rolled into one. But you know this duality of emotions by now. Your experiences will reflect it often and probably for the rest of your life. Don't try to suppress the emotions. Don't try to pretend they aren't there. Live them, experience them, survive them, and you will be okay.

There are countless ways you can honor the person you lost, and only you know what feels right. Maybe it's a race, a fund-raiser for a good cause, a hike to a mountaintop, or a visit to another country. As you continue down your individual road toward healing, you will realize that honoring them is as much, and more, about honoring yourself. You have chosen to live again because you are still here for a reason, and that is something to celebrate.

Anniversaries

One of the questions I get asked most frequently is "What do I do on *that* day?" and my response is always the same. Nobody can tell you what you should do, and I hope you listen to your heart and honor what feels right. That being said, on the anniversary of Mitch's accident I've always made the deliberate decision to do something from his bucket list. I try not to view the day as tragic and sad but rather as inspiring and hopeful, just like he lived his life. My Mitch was all about living, exploring, seeing, and doing, and I can't imagine he'd ever want his family to sit and waste a day of life. It's always been an easy choice for me, and the joy I experience living in his honor always overshadows the sorrow I feel in my heart for his passing.

An upcoming anniversary may throw you off for weeks or even months beforehand due to dread or trepidation. The anticipation is often worse than the day of the anniversary. Whatever you decide to do with that day, I hope you find some measure of peace. Throw a party with some friends, go for a hike up a quiet mountain, walk along the beach, listen to music, or write a poem. There is no right or wrong reaction to a difficult time. My theory for the day is my theory for all the other days you live beyond loss: forward movement is the greatest form of healing available. If you take an active step on that day, you can take two active steps tomorrow.

Spiritual Healing

Religion and spirituality may play a big role in your life after loss as well as your road toward healing. I encourage you to read, listen to others, and be open to the forms of spirituality that may serve you. I feel most spiritual when I sit on top of a mountain and gaze at all the beauty before me. Being indoors does not serve me in regards to my work, my play, or my spiritual life. Solitude, peace, and beauty connect me to my great consciousness and help me elevate my life in meaningful ways. Just like you have to figure out how your body works, you must also figure out how your mind works, how your emotions work, and how your forward path will work. Be willing to explore all the aspects of your personal growth as you evolve through the journey of grief.

Fitness and Nutrition Beyond 12 Weeks

Believe it or not, you've done the easy work so far. You've stayed on track for twelve weeks. Now it's time to remember that this is a life-long journey, and in order to stay the course you have to keep going. I will never forget when I completed my first bodybuilding competition. I was so lean, so fit, and so beyond what I ever thought I could be. I remember thinking *Well, that's it. I've arrived . . . I am* fit*!* and I allowed myself a moment of celebration. That's when I realized that if I didn't maintain my current work ethic in the gym and commitment to food in the kitchen, my fitness would fade. I was going to have to keep going, for *life.* Since that day, I've had countless highs and lows, and if I'm being honest, I have failed more than my fair share of times. I've missed workouts, picked poor foods, and beaten myself up. What I've learned is that each time I am not perfect I am given a chance in the very next moment to do and be better. Nobody is perfect all the time. What separates the people who will quit from the people who will fail and keep going is the basic understanding that a bump in the road is not the end of the line. Accept that failure, learn from it, and *immediately* get up and keep going! Don't allow your screw-ups to take you off course for life. Don't allow a bad day to turn into a bad life. If you find yourself off course, simply reevaluate your next move carefully and get back to LLAFP. Maybe you get in a walk, drink some extra water, or eat more veggies. Any action is better than no action at all. Remember how far you've come and get back to it. You've done much harder things in this life, and you can do this too.

Final Measurements and Fitness Test

Now that you have completed the Healthy Healing program, make sure you do your final measurements and take stock of your favorite non-scale victories to date. I also want you to revisit the fitness assessment we did at the beginning of the book and see how much stronger you have become. Sit with your success for a few minutes. Don't stress about how much further you think you could have gone; truly be proud of how far you did come. Whatever changes you made, whatever successes you had, it is an incredible accomplishment, and you should be very proud of your hard work. You made the hard choice to live your best life when you had every reason not to. I'm proud of you. You should be proud of yourself too.

	Week 1	Week 12
Air Squat:		
Mountain Climber:		
Push-Up:		
Plank:		

	Week 1	Week 6	Week 12
Neck:			
Chest:			
Arms:			
Waist:			
Hips:			
Quads:			
Calves:			

Rereading and Rewriting Your "Why"

Back at the beginning of your Healthy Healing journey I asked you to write yourself a "why" letter and keep it somewhere safe. Now I want you to revisit that letter and look at your "why" from twelve weeks ago. Take careful stock of what your "why" was then and how it has changed. Remember, you made all of those changes to reach your next level of living with nothing more than a bunch of baby steps strung together. You have baby-stepped your way toward a better life. Now it is time to write your "why" again and set your sights on newer and bigger goals for the next twelve weeks. Imagine where you can take yourself if you follow this pattern for years to come. You will become limitless, and all it takes is enough small steps forward.

Homework:
Carry Your Weight

Congratulations! You have come a long way in a short period of time. By taking small, daily baby steps, you have changed the course of your life in more ways than you probably even realize. Those daily baby steps are bigger and more difficult than we give them credit for. The last twelve weeks have shown you how to eat better, move better, and love life a little more. You've shed so much, both physically and emotionally. You've shed things that no longer serve you. You've shed some guilt, stress, and useless stuff, and perhaps even found some new happiness in your life after loss. You've purged your body of unwanted toxins, you've purged your mind of unnecessary guilt, and now it's time to remind yourself why all that extra weight is never worth carrying again. There is a real power in understanding how that weight feels.

This week's homework is designed to help you make that emotional and physical connection. I'd like you to add the weight you've lost over the past twelve weeks to a backpack and go for a one-mile walk. If weight loss was not your goal, you can still do this exercise by simply adding ten to fifteen pounds and labeling the weights with the emotional weight you have let go (for example, fear, anger, regret, and/or guilt). Head outside, into nature, and take a walk or a hike, using the time as a meditation in motion. Notice how the weight makes you feel, how it places pressure on your joints, your shoulders, your back, and your spirit. The walk will be challenging; carrying all that extra physical and emotional weight always takes its toll. Notice your breathing, the speed at which you move, and where your head is positioned during the mile. Is your breathing labored? Is your speed slow and heavy? Is your head looking down toward the ground?

After you've completed the mile, remove the weight and walk for a while longer, taking in the feeling after the weight is off your shoulders. Sense how much lighter your body feels—more importantly, how light your spirit feels. Has your breathing returned to normal? Do you walk faster and farther without the added baggage? Does your head come up and notice the beauty that surrounds you with each step? Are you looking forward instead of down?

The physical and emotional weight we carry can do untold damage to our bodies, our minds, and our spirits. It is important that we start to make this connection and release ourselves from the weight that holds us down. Remember, you didn't shed this weight in an hour or a day; you shed it over twelve weeks of hard work. You probably danced between the path forward and the path you left behind, sometimes taking steps back, only to push yourself forward again. Such is the path to fitness but also the path in life after loss. Dance until you find your pace comfortably on the path ahead. If you traveled this far in twelve weeks, just imagine where another year of baby steps will take you. If you surround yourself with the right community and keep fitness as your tool for life, you will become unstoppable in your forward progress.

I believe in you.

Please take photos of this homework and hashtag #healthyhealing if you post them, or share them on our interactive portal to let us know you're freeing yourself from the undue pressure of physical and emotional weight. I can't wait to see your head lifted and looking at the world around you.

Moving Forward Every Day

You've done some hard work over the past twelve weeks, and in many ways the fitness and nutrition was the easiest part. Compared to what you've lived with, what you've overcome, what you've survived, you can easily handle making the choice to live a full and fit life from this point forward. What's much harder is the choice to really live this life you have been given, because living beyond loss is never simple. While it's not the easy choice, I can tell that it's one you will never regret making—not only for yourself so much as for the lives of the people you love and the person you lost.

I won't ever tell you that life only hands you what you can handle, because frankly that's just not true. Life is going to hand you many things you don't think you can handle. But you won't ever tackle these challenges in one moment or in one step; rather, you will apply the concept of baby steps that you learned in this book for the remainder of your life. I want you to walk away from this program knowing that anything is possible and you have everything you need within you already. Turn to fitness on those harder-than-hard days, and never forget how alive it can make you feel to connect with your own strength. When your motivation wanes and you're struggling to do what you know will ultimately make you happier, dig deep within yourself and find that fire I know you have. Others may inspire you for a day or a week, but it's up to you to reconnect with your "why" and motivate yourself for the remainder of your life. Your "why" will change and grow, just like you, but if you never stop asking yourself the question, you won't ever run out of motivation.

I've spent the better part of this book giving you the tools necessary to use exercise, nutrition, and overall well-being for a healthier grief journey. What I've told you is backed by science, countless individuals who've chosen a similar path for healing, and of course my own experience. Regardless of all I've shared, it won't make a difference if you don't apply my words to your own life and decide to make a change for the better. There is only one person who can change your life, and that person is you. Regardless of what you've been through, regardless of what defines your past, only you can define the days that lie ahead. At some point you will need to come to terms with your loss and make the conscious decision to move forward. You will need to decide that you are not done writing your story, and as the author, you must pick up the pen and write again.

Let's go back to M. Scott Peck's words in *The Road Less Traveled:* "Life is difficult."

But our difficulties often prove to be our greatest life lessons, and the moments that define us are often our most challenging. This dawned on me when I was recently white-water rafting one of the ten best rivers in the Americas with one of My1FitLife's adventure groups in Costa Rica. As I sat there, catching my breath between the huge rapids, I took in the incredible beauty all around me, and my eyes welled up with tears.

My late husband loved to raft.

He loved nature.

He loved to live.

That moment was painful, sad, beautiful, inspiring, and difficult. That moment reminded me that my life would *forever* be full of duality. Grief leaves you with a new view of the world. It leaves you with the greatest appreciation for life and happiness, all while gutting you with anguish and pain. The duality is very real.

After a few moments on the raft, we all noticed the most beautiful blue butterfly following us, and I looked across at one of my fellow widows and saw tears in her eyes. She looked up at the butterfly and said, "There's my sign," and I could see the duality in her eyes so clearly. Joy and pain mixed exquisitely, like the waves of the mighty river. The butterfly followed our raft over the course of many miles, reminding us that while the people we loved are gone from our daily view, they are never truly far.

The duality of life after loss will forever remind you that the road is not flat or straight, but the best views always come after the hardest climbs.

I'm here to tell you, it's not over. This is not the end of your journey. It's just the beginning.

Throughout this process, you've seen that regardless of how tragic, how sad, and how horrifying life may be, you can reflect on life, ponder your circumstances, grieve, grow, and rest, and then pick up the pen and continue with the remainder of your story.

Never underestimate your strength, your bravery, or your power.

You are still here for a reason.

You should *live*.

—Michelle

Healthy Healing
Shopping List

PROTEINS

Almond or peanut butter

Beef (only occasionally), grass-fed and hormone-free

Chicken breast, organic, whole or ground

Eggs, organic

Fish (occasionally), especially salmon and halibut, wild-caught, fresh whenever possible

Legumes (beans, lentils, peas, etc.)

Nuts, raw and unsalted, especially almonds

Patties: beef, chicken, salmon, turkey, vegetable (select low-fat and chemical-free)

Seeds: chia, flax, pumpkin, sunflower, etc., raw and unsalted

Tuna, skipjack, packed in water

Turkey bacon (only occasionally)

Turkey breast, organic, whole, sliced, or ground

Turkey jerky

VEGETABLES

Arugula	Kale
Broccoli	Mushrooms
Brussels sprouts	Onions
Carrots	Romaine lettuce
Celery	Spinach
Garlic	Sweet peppers
Green beans	Sweet potatoes
Jicama	. . . and anything else local to you!

FRUITS

Apples	Limes
Avocados	Mangos
Bananas	Oranges
Berries, fresh or frozen	Tangerines
Lemons	

BEVERAGES, LIQUIDS

Almond milk	Coconut milk
Aloe vera juice	Coffee or espresso
Apple juice*	Teas, green and any other types
Carrot juice*	Vegetable juice*

*Prepare these beverages at home if possible.

SPICES AND HERBS
(FRESH WHENEVER POSSIBLE)

Arrowroot	Onion powder
Basil	Oregano
Chili powder and peppers	Parsley
Cinnamon	Pepper
Garlic powder	Saffron
Ginger	Sage
Mint	Tarragon
Nutmeg	Turmeric

BROTHS, CONDIMENTS, DIPS, OILS, VINEGARS

Avocado oil, organic

Broth, organic chicken

Coconut oil, cold-pressed, organic

Extra-virgin olive oil, organic

Hummus

Mustard

Homemade salsa

Vinegar, any variety

DRY FOODS

Barley

Beans, black and numerous other dried or canned types

Breads: Ezekiel sprouted whole grain or Dave's Killer Bread (preferably with 5 or fewer grams sugar)

Brown rice

Buckwheat groats

Cacao nibs, for baking

Lentils

Oats, steel cut or rolled

Popcorn, without butter

Quinoa

Split peas

SUPPLEMENTS (AS NEEDED)

Glucosamine, for joint support

L-Glutamine, for gut and immune-system function

Multivitamin

SWEETS

Applesauce

Chocolate, dark (preferably 70 or more percent cacao)

Coconut sugar

Dried fruit, unsweetened

Fresh fruit, preferably berries (refer to fruit list)

Stevia

Healthy Healing Recipes and Easy Meals

The following are just a few of my favorite fast and easy recipes. You can find more on the Healthy Healing website. When at all possible I recommend that you buy organic and fresh fruits and vegetables and preferably hormone-free, grass-fed, or organic meats and dairy products. The key is buying fresh and locally sourced products whenever possible and using as few ingredients in your cooking as necessary. Your road to health starts with good quality food—remember the food you eat makes up the cells of your body. Treat your body well and eat smart.

Michelle's Morning Smoothie

This is my absolute favorite morning smoothie. It serves just one and
is nutrient dense and refreshing.   *Serves 1*

8 to 16 ounces fresh organic spinach
1 medium banana
1 tablespoon fresh ginger
8 to 16 ounces almond, coconut, or rice milk
1 scoop organic green powder (optional; I use the brand Organifi,
   which can be found online)
Ice

Combine all the ingredients in a quality blender or Vitamix, and
puree until the mixture is smooth. Serve cold.

Banana Pancakes

No excuses with this recipe. It's fast, easy, and super good. The kids
will love it, and so will you. I make a big batch on Sunday and feed
my kids this one all week long. They go off to school with a solid mix
of protein, carbs, and good fat!   *Serves 2 to 4*

2 ripe bananas
4 eggs, or 6 egg whites
2 tablespoons peanut butter or almond butter
Dash of vanilla
Dash of ground cinnamon
1 cup oatmeal, uncooked (optional)
Coconut oil for the griddle

To make the batter, mix the bananas, eggs or egg whites, nut butter, vanilla, cinnamon, and optional oatmeal in a blender.

Heat the coconut oil on a griddle or in a sauté pan, and spoon the batter onto the heated surface for your pancakes, browning them lightly on both sides. They're a fantastic consistency and so sweet you don't even need syrup.

Grandma Mary's Oatmeal

This recipe is from Lorrie McFadden. You may include 2 whole eggs in the oatmeal—both egg whites and nutrient-rich yolks—or, to reduce fat, include just the whites, as the recipe states. *Serves 1*

1 cup organic traditional oats
1¾ cups water
Dash of salt
⅛ cup pecan pieces (optional)
2 egg whites
Fresh berries or half a banana
¼ cup almond milk

For creamy oatmeal, add the oats to the water and bring the combination to a boil in a saucepan. For chewy oatmeal, bring the water to a boil in a saucepan first, then add the oats. Reduce the heat to a simmer and cook the oats per the instructions provided with the product. Stir in the salt and the optional pecans.

When the oatmeal is 1 or 2 minutes from ready, rapidly stir in the egg whites and keep stirring rapidly for 1 minute, or until the egg whites are cooked through. For a creamy oatmeal with a minimal presence of egg whites, whisk the mixture immediately and quickly as you add the whites.

Serve with the fruit and the almond milk.

Bone Broth Potato Leek Soup

For the potatoes in this recipe, I use a combination of 4 Yukon Golds and 1 sweet potato. For the bone broth, you can make your own (or use chicken broth or vegetable stock), but I use Pacific brand (from Costco). And I love to use Himalayan salt in this soup. *Serves 4 to 6*

   2 tablespoons extra-virgin olive oil
   3 leeks, thinly sliced
   Salt and freshly ground black pepper to taste
   3 cloves garlic, minced
   5 medium potatoes, peeled and diced small
   3 cups bone broth
   3 cups almond or coconut milk, unsweetened

Optional Toppers

   1 tablespoon pico de gallo
   Pinch of crunchy bacon (baked or fried)
   Handful of freshly chopped Italian parsley

Heat the olive oil in a soup pot set over medium heat, and sauté the leeks in the oil, stirring them occasionally, for approximately 5 minutes, or until they are soft. Season your leeks to taste with salt and pepper. Add the minced garlic and simmer for about 30 seconds. (Don't overcook the garlic, or it will make the soup taste bitter.) Add the cubed potatoes and bone broth and bring them to a boil over medium-high heat. Cover the soup with a lid and let it cook for 10 to 12 minutes or until the potatoes are soft. Add the unsweetened almond or coconut milk (less or more depending on how thick you like your soup). Transfer the soup to a mixer, Vitamix, or other blender, or you can use an immersion blender in the pot on the stove. Puree until the soup is smooth. Add more salt and pepper as needed and top with one or all of the delicious options above.

Salmon Salad with Balsamic Dressing

Need dinner in 15 minutes? Have a salad that's fast, nutritious, and delicious. While this makes a refreshing summer salad, smoked salmon works into the fall and beyond. If you can't find fresh berries, change it up with avocado, pomegranate seeds, cranberries, or even the sweeter mango or pineapple. The sweeter the fruit, the lighter the dressing! Go with whatever is in season. *Serves 6 to 8*

24 to 32 ounces fresh organic mixed greens
24 to 32 cups fresh organic baby spinach
½ pound smoked salmon, pulled into bite-size pieces
⅓ cup chopped red bell pepper
¼ cup chopped red onion
1 teaspoon dijon mustard
1 teaspoon vinegar
2 tablespoons extra-virgin olive oil
1 clove garlic, minced
¼ teaspoon black pepper
Salt to taste (optional)
¾ cup fresh berries

In a serving bowl, combine the greens and spinach with the salmon, red bell pepper, and onion. Set the salad aside.

For the dressing, in a jar or a small bowl, combine the dijon mustard, vinegar, olive oil, garlic, black pepper, and optional salt, then either shake the jar vigorously or whisk the ingredients in the bowl until the vinaigrette is well blended.

Drizzle the dressing over the salad, lightly toss until everything is coated, then top the salad with the berries.

Pistachio Spinach Salad

This is one of my all-time favorite salads. It's full of nutrients and tastes *amazing*. You simply can't go wrong with this flavor combination. Put it together in about 15 minutes and enjoy!   *Serves 6 to 8*

32 to 64 ounces fresh organic spinach
½ cup quinoa, cooked and cooled completely
8 ounces roasted and chopped pistachios
½ cup extra-virgin olive oil, or to taste
Juice of 2 lemons
Dash of sea salt
Dash of black pepper
Small pinch of red pepper flakes
¼ cup goat or feta cheese

Wash and dry the spinach, place it in a large salad bowl, and toss it together with the quinoa and the pistachios. Set the salad aside.

In a small bowl, whisk together the olive oil, lemon juice, salt, black pepper, and red pepper flakes. Drizzle the dressing over the salad, coating everything well.

Top the salad with the cheese and serve immediately.

Kid-Approved Spinach Smoothie

My kids love sweet smoothies, and I love getting as much spinach in their lives as possible. This one has all kinds of goodness inside, and they can't drink it fast enough! Besides the spinach, which is so good for their health, the smoothie is packed with antioxidants (berries, chia seeds), omega-3s (chia seeds), fiber (chia seeds), and protein (goat yogurt, chia seeds). I'm allergic to cow's milk, so we use lots of alternatives in our home. Goat yogurt is very easy to digest, but you can also use Greek yogurt. Avoid anything other than plain yogurt, though. Flavored yogurts are full of added and unnecessary sugars.

Serves 2

16 ounces fresh organic spinach, well washed
1 cup plain goat yogurt
½ apple
1 banana
1 cup frozen berries (raspberries, blueberries, and/or strawberries)
2 tablespoons chia seeds

In a high-quality blender or Vitamix, place the spinach, then the goat yogurt, then the apple and the banana. Add to this combination the frozen berries. Top with the chia seeds, then blend the mixture until it's smooth. Serve cold.

Santa Fe Turkey Burger

For lean and mean burgers that you can make in minutes, this recipe from Lorrie McFadden hits the spot. I make my own salsa and cover it, but you can go as easy or as heavy as you like. It goes great with sweet potato fries on the side and extra salsa for dipping (no catsup needed)! Use high-quality organic turkey for your burgers for a much more flavorful and healthy meal. Choose a favorite salsa or make your own. It's quite easy.   *Serves 4 to 6*

12 ounces ground turkey or chicken
¾ cup diced red bell pepper
¼ cup diced sweet onion, or 1½ tablespoons onion powder
¾ teaspoon ground or leaf oregano
¼ teaspoon cayenne pepper
¾ teaspoon ground cumin
½ teaspoon garlic powder
Salt and black pepper to taste
Whole-wheat buns (optional)
½ cup salsa
1 medium avocado, sliced
8 ounces fresh organic spring mix greens

In a bowl, mix together by hand the ground meat, red bell pepper, onion or onion powder, oregano, cayenne, cumin, garlic powder, salt, and pepper. Knead until all the ingredients are well combined, then form patties of your desired size.

Grill the patties or cook them in a sauté pan until they are cooked through, approximately 10 minutes.

Serve the patties hot on whole-wheat buns (if desired) topped with your favorite salsa, the sliced avocado, and salad greens.

Quick and Easy Hummus

This hummus from Lorrie McFadden makes a great dip served with celery, carrots, and red bell peppers. It also makes a wonderful spread, adding protein, texture, and flavor to an otherwise uninspired sandwich! *Serves 2 to 4*

15.5-ounce can garbanzo beans, drained and juice reserved
¼ cup juice from garbanzo bean can
1 clove garlic, chopped
Juice of ⅓ large lemon, or to taste
1 tablespoon tahini
⅛ teaspoon salt, or to taste
¼ teaspoon black pepper
1 tablespoon extra-virgin olive oil
Paprika (optional)

Puree all the ingredients in a quality blender. Serve the hummus in a decorative bowl with additional olive oil drizzled over the top, or use it as a spread.

Lemony Vinaigrette

Lorrie McFadden contributed this yummy dressing too. It's great on salads or steamed vegetables.

¼ cup extra-virgin olive oil
¼ cup apple cider vinegar
3 tablespoons freshly squeezed lemon juice
Zest of 1 small lemon
1½ tablespoons coconut sugar

Put all the ingredients in a jar, a small bowl, or a food processor, and shake, whisk, or process the mixture until it is well combined. Store any extra in the refrigerator in a small mason jar with a lid. It will last several weeks.

Acknowledgments

Writing this book has been a tremendous undertaking. Everyone tells you how complicated the process is, but I did not understand until I jumped in with both feet and found myself overwhelmed with the process. There are countless people I'd like to thank for their love, advice, patience, dedication, and acceptance because truth be told, I'd still be on my message to the reader without them.

These thank-yous are in no particular order because each person has touched my life and made me smile during this daunting process.

My amazing tribe at My1FitLife, One Fit Widow, and Live the List

What can I say about the people who have become like family to me over the years? My Fitness "Questies" who have pushed me forward and become my biggest cheerleaders through this process! To those who kindly follow and participate at One Fit Widow, who have brought me so much joy and happiness, I'm thankful for each one of you. When you tell me you've chosen to live again after loss, you make each day worth it. The incredible people at Live the List—and especially Lisa Shaw Marotto who helped to bring my vision to life—you inspire me deeply.

My Friends and Family

I have a large family, and I'm blessed with some pretty amazing friends. I won't list everyone, but I'm deeply thankful to you all for your continued love and support.

Lynn Lancaster

Lynn helped guide me through the book proposal process and countless revisions and do-overs. She helped steer me and my writing to a home with HarperCollins. I'm thankful for her good editing eye and sweet friendship. I wouldn't be here without her.

Christina Rasmussen

My widow sister and fellow advocate for life after loss. Christina has been a fierce and loyal friend since I started One Fit Widow, as well as a dedicated mentor and fellow author. There are days, without her encouragement, that I may have quit because it all became too much. She reminds me that my mission is one worth fighting for.

Mel and Barbara Berger

This book would have never seen the light of day without the help of my agent Mel Berger. When Mel and I first spoke, I was intimidated and overwhelmed, but he helped me feel at ease with the process and efficiently brought my work to the right people. Mel's wife was my silent cheerleader, and while I've never corresponded with her, he assures me she is the reason I've been blessed with this relationship. For that, I am forever thankful to them both.

Hilary Lawson

My amazing and patient editor at HarperCollins who held my hand, made me feel better (all the time), and kept me going in the right direction. Hilary is a fierce advocate for strong female voices, and our world could use many more women lifting one another up just as Hilary has done for me. Thank you, Hilary, for a year-plus of your life holding my hand through this process.

My editing and marketing team at HarperCollins

Amazing, smart, and fun people. I'm deeply indebted to this entire team who has brought Healthy Healing to light. I feel blessed to be in your care.

Gary and Thu Steinke

My late husband's parents, who have been my rock over nearly the past eight years. There are not enough words to describe just how special they are to my kids and me. Their love and dedication to not only their grandchildren, but to their son's wife, is nothing short of incredible. I love them deeply, and I'm blessed to call them family.

Christine Appleton, Amy Price, and Kris Kobza

My closest friends who stood by me after my loss and never walked away. These three women have seen me through so much, and I owe them more than I can say. In all these years, they have never once complained about my grief, they have never asked me to stop talking about him, and they have always honored his life and his love. Friends like this are hard to find, and I'm lucky to call these women my sisters.

Lorrie McFadden

My sister who flew to my side on that devastating day and has never left since. Lorrie is a big part of what we do at One Fit Widow and My1FitLife, and her love and compassion for others is unparalleled. I'm so thankful for her presence in my life.

Quentin Gessner

My father, who in many ways has inspired most of the wisdom throughout this book. He shared with me his love of nature, fitness, and living, so I can, in turn, share it with all of you.

My children: Haven, Kane, Addison, and Matthew

So much of what I do begins and ends with my kids. I hope they learn from me the beauty of life and the importance of choice. These four inspire me to be better, and without their support and understanding during the year it took to write this book, it would have never come to be. I love you all deeply; you are my greatest accomplishment.

Keith Baumgard, My Man Who Came After

I said this was in no particular order but when it comes to Keith . . . that's a lie. Since coming into my life, Keith has been an incredible force. Keith's patience, deep love, and understanding never cease to amaze me. Without Keith, this book would still be just a dream in my head. His shared passion for fitness and for helping others has been a key component of how I got this far. Keith, you are loved deeply, and I can't wait to share the road ahead with you.

Resources

Some of My Personal Favorite Books

The Code of the Extraordinary Mind by Vishen Lakhiani (New York: Simon and Schuster, 2016)

Exercise for Mood and Anxiety by Michael W. Otto and Jasper A. J. Smits (New York: Oxford University Press, 2011)

The Fifth Agreement by Don Miguel Ruiz and Don José Ruiz (San Rafael, CA: Amber-Allen, 2010)

Finding Your Way After Your Spouse Dies by Marta Felber (Notre Dame, IN: Ava Maria Press, 2008)

The Four Agreements by Don Miguel Ruiz (San Rafael, CA: Amber-Allen, 2010)

The Grief Recovery Handbook by John W. James and Russell Friedman (New York: HarperCollins, 2009)

The Happiness Advantage by Shawn Achor (New York: Broadway Books, 2010)

Head Strong by Dave Asprey (New York: HarperCollins, 2017)

The Healing Power of Exercise by Linn Goldberg and Diane L. Elliot (New York: John Wiley and Sons, 2000)

I'm Grieving as Fast as I Can by Linda Feinberg (New York: New Horizon Press, 2013)

I Wasn't Ready to Say Goodbye by Brook Noel and Pamela Blair (Naperville, IL: Sourcebooks, 2008)

The Mastery of Love by Don Miguel Ruiz (White Plains, NY: Peter Pauper Press, 2004)

The Miracle Morning by Hal Elrod (Temecula, CA: Hal Elrod International, 2016)

The Road Less Traveled by M. Scott Peck (New York: Touchstone, 1993)

Second Firsts by Christina Rasmussen (Carlsbad, CA: Hay House, 2013)

Spark by John J. Ratey and Eric Hagerman (Boston: Little, Brown, 2008)

When Bad Things Happen to Good People by Harold S. Kushner (New York: Schocken Books, 2001)

Widow to Widow by Genevieve Davis Ginsburg (Tucson, AZ: Fisher Books, 1997)

The Year of Magical Thinking by Joan Didion (New York: Vintage Books, 2007)

You Are a Badass by Jen Sincero (Philadelphia: Running Press, 2013)

Healthy Healing Online Resources

For useful grief community resources, see my nonprofit, Live the List:
www.livethelistnonprofit.org.

You can reach out to our fitness community at www.my1fitlife.com.

You can find more information about all topics covered in this book, including
additional recipes, workouts, and other resources, at our online interactive
portal: www.healthyhealingbook.com/healing.

Other Online Resources

Alliance of Hope

http://www.allianceofhope.org

The Alliance of Hope for Suicide Loss Survivors provides healing support
for people coping with the shock, excruciating grief, and complex emotions
that accompany the loss of a loved one to suicide.

American Widow Project

http://americanwidowproject.org

The mission of the American Widow Project is to provide military widows
with vital support through peer-based programs designed to educate,
empower, inspire, and assist them in rebuilding their lives in the face of
tragedy.

A2Z Healing Toolbox

http://www.a2zhealingtoolbox.com

Susan Hannifin-MacNab is a social worker, educator, and community
organizer who has spent the last twenty years teaching and leading "health
and wellness" workshops, classes, and support groups for youth and families
on the mainland of the United States, Canada, and Australia. After the
sudden, traumatic death of her husband in 2012, Susan's life took an
unexpected turn into the world of grief, loss, and trauma—and ultimately,
post-traumatic growth and continued healing.

Camp Widow

http://www.campwidow.org

Camp Widow is a weekend-long gathering of widowed people from
across the country and around the world who come together to create a
community that understands the life-altering experience of widowhood.
Camp Widow provides practical tools, valuable resources, and peer-based

encouragement for rebuilding your life in the aftermath of the death of a spouse . . . all in a fun, uplifting, laughter-filled atmosphere.

Concerns of Police Survivors (COPS)

http://www.nationalcops.org

COPS was organized in 1984 with 110 individual members. Today COPS membership is over 37,000 survivors, including spouses, children, parents, siblings, significant others, and affected coworkers of officers killed in the line of duty according to federal government criteria. COPS is governed by a national board of law enforcement survivors. All programs and services are administered by the national office in Camdenton, Missouri. COPS has more than fifty chapters nationwide that work with survivors at the grass-roots level.

Gary Roe

http://www.garyroe.com/

Writer, chaplain, and grief counselor Gary Roe provides a range of resources on grief and healing on his website, including the Good Grief mini course that some of our members have benefitted from.

Grief Share

http://www.griefshare.org

Grief Share is a friendly, caring group of people who will walk alongside you through one of life's most difficult experiences. You don't have to go through the grieving process alone.

Live the List

http://www.livethelistnonprofit.org

"Helping others live big or small dreams for their best life after loss."

Live the List (my nonprofit) is making a difference in the lives of widows, widowers, and their children. It helps individuals lead by example and positively shape generations after a devastating loss. As the organization states, we can all do great things, but sometimes we need the help, encouragement, and financial support of others to make great things happen.

Do you have a dream to fulfill that will put your life on the right path? A goal—big or small—that will help you live a purposeful life and live the list? Apply for sponsorship and let Live the List help move you forward.

Modern Widows Club

http://modernwidowsclub.com

This is a widow-mentoring organization that inspires widows to live a life in which anything is possible. The organization does this by being a friend and mentor and by advocating in the widows' favor. It holds kindness, compassion, and James 1:27 to heart, moving forward while reaching back.

National Hospice and Palliative Care Organization

http://www.nhpco.org

If your spouse or partner is/was involved in hospice, this organization offers up to one year of free grief counseling. They also offer community outreach counseling for people whose spouse or partner was not in hospice but who still need grief counseling. Finally, if the counseling offered does not meet your needs, contact the bereavement department of your local hospice; they are usually happy to help you locate local grief services and support that is more appropriate for you.

Second Firsts

http://www.secondfirsts.com

Second Firsts was founded in 2010 by crisis-intervention counselor and author Christina Rasmussen. It provides a scientific and process-oriented approach to releasing pain consciously and methodically by relying on the brain's ability to give birth to new pathways, habits, and brain connections.

Soaring Spirits International

www.soaringspirits.org

Soaring Spirits is an inclusive, nondenominational organization focused on hope and healing through the grieving process. It is positive and forward thinking, while focusing on offering its members the tools and resources they need to rebuild their lives in the aftermath of the death of a loved one.

Support After Suicide

http://supportaftersuicide.org.uk

Support After Suicide is a partnership of organizations that provides bereavement support in the UK.

Tragedy Assistance Program for Survivors (TAPS)

http://www.taps.org/

TAPS offers grief resources and bereavement counseling to those grieving the loss of a loved one who served in the armed forces. Transition services, counseling, and outreach are provided through a national peer support network at no cost to surviving families and loved ones. The organization also partners with the U.S. Department of Veterans Affairs.

Widowed Village
http://widowedvillage.org

Widowed Village—a program of Soaring Spirits International—connects peers for friendship and sharing. The moderators, administrators, and others involved in running this site are widowed people like you. Peer support is an excellent, social way to learn more about living with loss while gaining the energy and ideas for your path to a new life.

Young Widow Forum
http://widda.org

The Young Widow Forum is a moderated online community that exists to help the young widowed to recover, reclaim, and rebuild by facilitating the exchange of experiences, information, and support. The forum offers opportunities to share your story and relate to others who share similar experiences. Sections of the board include general topics, timeline (topics based on the time since your loss), specific circumstances (topics based on whether or not you have children; on whether your relationship was affected by suicide, addiction, mental illness, or domestic violence; on extreme caregiving; etc.), socializing, and encouragement.

Psychological Support

American Psychological Association (APA) Online Help Center
http://www.apa.org/helpcenter/

APA's Psychology Help Center is an online consumer resource featuring articles and information related to psychological issues affecting your daily physical and emotional well-being. The website has a number of online resources, including a tool to look up psychological support and counseling in your area.

National Suicide Prevention Lifeline
http://www.suicidepreventionlifeline.org/
1-800-273-TALK (8255)

If you feel you are in a crisis, whether or not you are thinking about killing yourself, please call the Suicide Prevention Lifeline. People have called the lifeline for help with substance abuse, economic worries, relationship and family problems, sexual orientation, illness, getting over abuse, depression, mental and physical illness, and even loneliness.

When you dial 1-800-273-TALK (8255), you are calling the crisis center in the Lifeline network closest to your location. When you call, you will hear a message saying you have reached the National Suicide Prevention Lifeline, then hold music while your call is routed to the appropriate location. You will be helped by a skilled, trained crisis worker who will listen to your problems and tell you about mental health services in your area. Your call is confidential and free.

Parenting and Supporting Grieving Children

New Song Center for Grieving Children—Arizona Only

http://www.hov.org/welcome-new-song-center-grieving-children

This program of Hospice of the Valley offers grief support group experiences for children, teens, young adults, and their family caregivers following the death of a loved one. New Song creates a safe place in which children engage in developmentally appropriate activities, including art, play, and journaling. Adults attend their own support groups, where they learn how to help children process grief in a healthy manner and how to help themselves cope with loss. The center also provides grief education for caregivers, community groups, schools, clergy, and medical and mental health professionals. Services are all provided at no cost to the participants.

Stepping Stones of Hope

http://steppingstonesofhope.org

This organization's programs provide support for grieving families to help bereaved children become healthy, well-adjusted adults who may learn skills to navigate their own grief journeys as well as build family cohesion.

Grief Camps for Children

A grief camp is a great way for kids to learn about grief and to realize they are not alone. Many camps teach kids about grief as well as educate parents about how kids grieve differently than adults. The following are examples of grief camps held in several states; however, if you don't see one in your state, it is definitely worth doing a search online.

Camp Courage

http://www.bereavementcamp.org

The mission of the Camp Courage bereavement camps and the Pre-Camp Grief Support Group is to facilitate the grieving process of children, teens, and their families who have suffered the death of a significant person, while providing a safe and healing experience.

Camp Hometown Heroes

http://www.hometownheroes.org/

Camp Hometown Heroes is a national *free* weeklong overnight summer camp for children and siblings between the ages of seven and seventeen of fallen U.S. service members who died in any manner: combat, accident, illness, or suicide. During their visit to camp, perhaps for the first time in their young lives, the children have the opportunity to openly discuss their feelings and experiences. Through the support of pediatric grief specialists, the children partake in art and music therapy programs and optional discussion groups.

Comfort Zone Camp

http://www.comfortzonecamp.org

Comfort Zone Camp is a nonprofit 501(c)(3) bereavement camp that transforms the lives of children who have experienced the death of a parent, sibling, or legal guardian. The free camps include confidence-building programs and age-based support groups that break the emotional isolation grief often brings. Comfort Zone Camp is offered to children from seven to seventeen years old and is held year-round across the country. The nonprofit has offices in California, Massachusetts, New Jersey, and Virginia.

The Moyer Foundation

http://www.moyerfoundation.org

The mission of the Moyer Foundation is to provide comfort, hope, and healing to children and families affected by grief and addiction. Its innovative resources and programs address the critical needs of children experiencing powerful, overwhelming, and often confusing emotions associated with the death of someone close to them or substance abuse in their family. No child should have to face these struggles alone, and the foundation's unique programs bring kids together to ease their pain and provide the tools to help restore hope.

Stepping Stones of Hope (Camp Paz)—Arizona Only

http://www.steppingstonesofhope.org

This is only one of the camps the Stepping Stones of Hope organization offers. Through art, music, role-playing, and a lot of talking and laughing, kids learn about death and dying. And they learn how to begin to cope. At the same time, nearby and in a separate location, adult family members explore their grief through journaling, music, art, self-care, relaxation, and dialogue. Plus, they discover ways to best support the children who share their loss.

Notes

Message to the Reader

1. M. Scott Peck M.D., *The Road Less Traveled: A New Psychology of Love, Traditional Values and Spiritual Growth* (New York: Simon & Schuster, 1979).

Chapter 1: Myths About Grief

1. Michelle E. Steinke, "Stifled Grief: How the West Has It Wrong," *Healthy Living* [blog], *Huffington Post,* June 3, 2016, www.huffingtonpost.com /michelle-e-steinke/stifled-grief-how-the-wes_b_10243026.html.
2. Michelle E. Steinke, "Dear Widow Police—I Won't Revoke My Card," *One Fit Widow,* August 20, 2015, http://www.onefitwidow.com/blog/post /dear-widow-police--i-wont-revoke-my-card.
3. Christina Rasmussen, *Second Firsts: Live, Laugh and Love Again* (Carlsbad, CA: Hay House, November 4, 2013).
4. Michelle E. Steinke, "Widowhood: The Glass House of Grief," *One Fit Widow,* September 5, 2015, http://www.onefitwidow.com/blog/post /widowhood-the-glass-house-of-grief.
5. Lorna Collier, "Growth After Trauma: Why Are Some People More Resilient Than Others and Can It Be Taught," *Monitor on Psychology* 47, no. 10 (2016): 48, http://www.apa.org/monitor/2016/11/growth -trauma.aspx.

Chapter 2: Your Grief on Endorphins

1. John J. Ratey and Eric Hagerman, *Spark: The Revolutionary New Science of Exercise and the Brain* (Boston: Little, Brown, 2008).
2. Ratey and Hagerman, *Spark.*
3. Ratey and Hagerman, *Spark.*
4. "Depression," Fact Sheet, World Health Organization, last modified February 2017, http://www.who.int/mediacentre/factsheets/fs369/en/.
5. "Mental Health: Depression," Centers for Disease Control and Prevention, last modified March 30, 2016, https://www.cdc.gov/mentalhealth/basics /mental-illness/depression.htm.

6. Linn Goldberg, M.D. and Diane L. Elliot, M.D., *The Healing Power of Exercise: Your Guide to Preventing and Treating Diabetes, Depression, Heart Disease, High Blood Pressure, Arthritis, and More* (Canada: John Wiley and Sons, Inc. 2000).

7. "What Causes Depression?" Harvard Health Publications, Harvard Medical School, June 2009, www.health.harvard.edu/mind-and-mood /what-causes-depression.

8. Christopher Bergland, "25 Studies Confirm: Exercise Prevents Depression," *The Athlete's Way* [blog], *Psychology Today,* October 29, 2013, https:// www.psychologytoday.com/blog/the-athletes-way/201310/25-studies -confirm-exercise-prevents-depression.

9. "Anxiety," *Merriam-Webster,* https://www.merriam-webster.com/dictionary /anxiety.

10. "Post-Traumatic Stress Disorder (PTSD)," Diseases & Conditions, Mayo Clinic, February 2017, www.mayoclinic.org/diseases-conditions/post -traumatic-stress-disorder/home/ovc-20308548.

11. Matthew Tull, "The Benefits of Exercise for People with PTSD," Verywell, February 15, 2017, https://www.verywell.com/exercise -for-ptsd-2797465.

12. "How Does Exercise Help Those with Chronic Insomnia?" Ask the Expert, National Sleep Foundation, https://sleepfoundation.org/ask-the -expert/how-does-exercise-help-those-chronic-insomnia.

Chapter 3: Exercise

1. "What Is Pilates?" Pilates Fitness Institute, http://www.pfiwa.com.au/start /what-is-pilates.

2. G. N. Bratman, J. P. Hamilton, K. S. Hahn, G. C. Daily, and J. J. Gross, "Nature Experience Reduces Rumination and Subgenual Prefrontal Cortex Activation," *Proceedings of the National Academy of Sciences of the United States* 112, no. 28 (2015): 8567–72, www.pnas.org/content/112/28 /8567.abstract.

3. Dr. Mercola, "The Effects of Grounding," Mercola.com, November 21, 2015, http://articles.mercola.com/sites/articles/archive/2015/11/21 /grounding-effects.aspx.

4. Megan Ware, "Vitamin D: Health Benefits, Facts, and Research," *Medical News Today,* April 7, 2016, http://www.medicalnewstoday.com/articles /161618.php.

5. Rachel Nall, "Additional Sunlight Benefits," Healthline.com, November 9, 2015, www.healthline.com/health/depression /benefits-sunlight#benefits3.

Chapter 4: Nutrition

1. Colleen Pierre, "15 Mood-Boosting Foods," Health: Natural Remedies, *Prevention,* November 3, 2011, http://www.prevention.com/health/food-and-mood-best-foods-make-you-feel-better.

2. "Antioxidants and Free Radicals," SportsMedWeb, June 1996, http://www.rice.edu/~jenky/sports/antiox.html.

3. "Beta-Carotene," MedlinePlus, U.S. National Library of Medicine, June 3, 2015, www.nlm.nih.gov/medlineplus/druginfo/natural/999.html.

4. Emily Deans, "Do Carbs Keep You Sane?" *Psychology Today,* March 11, 2012, www.psychologytoday.com/blog/evolutionary-psychiatry/201203/do-carbs-keep-you-sane.

5. Susan Biali, "How Food Can Improve Your Mood," *Psychology Today,* July 29, 2009, www.psychologytoday.com/blog/prescriptions-life/200907/how-food-can-improve-your-moods.

6. A. Coppen and C. Bolander-Gouaille, "Treatment of Depression: Time to Consider Folic Acid and Vitamin B12," Abstract, *Journal of Psychopharmacology* 19, no. 1 (2005): www.ncbi.nlm.nih.gov/pubmed/15671130.

7. Dave Asprey, *Head Strong: The Bulletproof Plan to Activate Brain Energy to Work Smarter and Faster—in Just Two Weeks* (New York: HarperCollins, 2017).

8. Amy Paturel, "Brain Power with Good Fats," Cleveland Clinic Wellness, September 8, 2009, www.clevelandclinicwellness.com/food/GoodFats/Pages/BoostBrainPowerwithGoodFats.aspx.

9. "Mood Altering Foods," PGHUSA, *Never Stop Learning Ever,* October 6, 2006, http://neverstoplearningever.blogspot.com/2006/10/.

10. Larry Christensen and Ross Burrows, "Dietary Treatment of Depression," *Behavior Therapy* 21 (1990): 183-193, http:www.naturalstresscare.org/Media/Christensen_1990.pdf.

11. James Schend, "15 Foods That Boost the Immune System," *Healthline,* March 16, 2017, http://www.healthline.com/health/food-nutrition/foods-that-boost-the-immune-system#overview1.

12. M. S. Butt, M. T. Sultan, and J. Iqbal, "Garlic: Nature's Protection Against Physiological Threats," *Critical Reviews in Food Science and Nutrition* 49, no. 6 (2009): 538–51, http://www.ncbi.nlm.nih.gov/pubmed/19484634.

13. R. Alizadeh-Navaei, F. Roozbeh, M. Saravi, M. Pouramir, F. Jalali, and A. A. Moghadamnia, "Investigation of the Effect of Ginger on the Lipid Levels: A Double Blind Controlled Clinical Trial," *Saudi Medical Journal* 29, no. 9 (2008): 1280–84, http://www.smj.org.sa/index.php/smj/article/view/6361; and A. S. Al-Noory, A. N. Amreen, and S. Hymoor, "Antihyperlipidemic Effects of Ginger Extracts in Alloxan-Induced Diabetes and Propylthiouracil-Induced Hypothyroidism in (Rats)," Abstract,

Pharmacognosy Research 5, no. 3 (2013): 157–61, http://www.ncbi.nlm.nih
.gov/pubmed/23901210.

14. S. N. Meydani and W. K. Ha, "Immunologic Effects of Yogurt," *American
Journal of Clinical Nutrition* 71, no. 4 (2000): 861–72, https://www.ncbi.nlm
.nih.gov/pubmed/10731490.

Week 1: Time Management

1. Lorrie McFadden, "Ingredient Watch!" My1FitLife, https://1fwtraining
.com/nutrition/what-should-i-eat/ingredient-watch/.

Week 2: Guilt

1. Zig Ziglar, "Your Altitude," Ziglar.com, August 2, 2015, https://
www.ziglar.com/quotes/your-attitude-not-your-aptitude/.

2. Shawn Achor, *The Happiness Advantage: The Seven Principles of Positive
Psychology That Fuel Success and Performance at Work* (New York: Crown
Business, 2010).

Week 4: Comparison

1. Stephanie Dutchen, "What Do Fats Do in the Body?" *LiveScience,*
December 15, 2010, http://www.livescience.com/9109-fats-body.html.

2. "The Truth About Fats: The Good, the Bad, and the In Between," Harvard
Health Publications, Harvard Medical School, February 2015, www.health
.harvard.edu/staying-healthy/the-truth-about-fats-bad-and-good.

Week 5: Rest

1. Yvette Brazier, "Sleep Well to Avoid Insulin Resistance," *Medical News
Today,* November 4, 2015, http://www.medicalnewstoday.com/articles
/301721.php.

Week 6: A New Normal

1. Christina Rasmussen, *Second Firsts: Live, Laugh and Love Again* (Carlsbad,
CA: Hay House, November 4, 2013).

Week 7: Community

1. J. Holt-Lunstad, T. B. Smith, M. Baker, T. Harris, and D. Stephenson,
"Loneliness and Social Isolation as Risk Factors for Mortality," *SAGE* 10,
no. 2 (2015): 227–37, http://journals.sagepub.com/doi/full/10.1177
/1745691614568352.

Week 8: Numbing the Pain

1. Pete McCall, "7 Things to Know About Excess Post-Exercise Oxygen Consumption (EPOC)," *American Council on Exercise,* August 28, 2014, https://www.acefitness.org/blog/5008/7-things-to-know-about-excess -post-exercise-oxygen.
2. McCall, "7 Things to Know About Excess Post-Exercise Oxygen Consumption (EPOC)."
3. Dave Asprey, *Head Strong: The Bulletproof Plan to Activate Brain Energy to Work Smarter and Faster—in Just Two Weeks* (New York: HarperCollins, 2017).

Week 9: Planning for the Future

1. Vishen Lakhiani, *The Code of the Extraordinary Mind: 10 Unconventional Laws to Redefine Your Life and Succeed on Your Own Terms* (New York: Rodale Books, 2016).

Week 10: Leading by Example

1. Lorrie McFadden, "Eating Clean on a Budget," Living Fit, My1FitLife, December 14, 2013, https://1fwtraining.com/eating-clean-on-a-budget/.
2. "Dirty Dozen," Environmental Working Group, 2017, https://www.ewg .org/foodnews/dirty_dozen_list.php.
3. "Clean Fifteen," Environmental Working Group, 2017, https://www.ewg .org/foodnews/clean_fifteen_list.php.

Index

About the Author

MICHELLE STEINKE-BAUMGARD is a mother, remarried widow, IFPA certified personal trainer, and IFPA certified sports nutrition specialist. After losing her husband Mitch in 2009, she turned to exercise as an outlet for grief and a way to handle stress. Michelle found it so powerful that she eventually quit her corporate vice-president job to become a fitness coach. Since then Michelle has been featured in *Fitness, Shape,* and *Woman's World* and has contributed articles to *Prevention,* the *Huffington Post,* and countless other media outlets. As cofounder of One Fit Widow, My1FitLife, and Live the List, Michelle is focused on helping widows and widowers complete bucket list dreams to honor their late spouses while moving boldly into their futures. Michelle's overarching goal is to help people live a full, fit, and intentional life beyond life's hardest moments. She lives in Montana with her family.